DMSO

To the many scientists all over the world who have made contributions to an understanding of the chemistry and biology of DMSO

DMSO

The True Story of a Remarkable Pain-killing Drug

BARRY TARSHIS
from the exclusive files of
Dr. Stanley Jacob
and
Robert Herschler

WILLIAM MORROW AND COMPANY, INC.
New York   1981

The author and publisher wish to note that DMSO, the subject of this book, has not been legalized for use by all states. Readers should in no event use the drug without consulting their physician.

Produced by Engel & Engel

Library of Congress Cataloging in Publication Data

Tarshis, Barry.
    DMSO, the true story of a remarkable pain-killing drug.

        Bibliography: p.
        Includes index.
        1. Dimethyl sulphoxide. 2. Dimethyl sulphoxide
—History. I. Jacob, Stanley W. II. Herschler,
Robert. III. Title.
RM666.D56T37   615′.783   81-11343
ISBN 0-688-00716-3   AACR2

Printed in the United States of America

First Edition

1   2   3   4   5   6   7   8   9   10

BOOK DESIGN BY MICHAEL MAUCERI

Foreword

DMSO is not an easy subject to talk about unemotionally —least of all for the two of us. We believed when we first discovered the medical applications of DMSO that we had uncovered a substance more broadly useful in fighting disease than any other drug known to man, including aspirin. And we are firmer in this conviction today, nearly eighteen years later, than we have ever been before. We've witnessed the relief that DMSO has brought to thousands of people—people who, in many instances, had all but given up hope that they would ever live normal lives again. In our collective libraries are thousands of scientific studies, clinical reports and personal correspondence from scientists from all over the world that dramatically reinforce our convictions. We know that DMSO is both a safe and useful drug, and we know that for certain conditions— certain types of injuries and certain types of pain— DMSO is a more effective treatment than any other drug now in use. We also believe—and the belief carries with it a considerable amount of anguish and sorrow—that millions of people are suffering needlessly today—and in some cases dying—because after eighteen years DMSO is as yet unavailable to the average person through normal medical channels.

We hope this book will help to bring about a change in this unconscionable state of affairs. We agreed to open our files to Barry Tarshis, the author of this book, because so much of what has been written about DMSO in the lay press over the past eighteen years has presented a distorted picture of what DMSO is, how it works and why it has taken the Food and Drug Administration so long to make it accessible to the people whose lives could be immeasurably improved if DMSO were made available to them. We think this book serves a crucial need, for it presents for the first time the *true* story of DMSO.

What you read in this book is likely to encourage you, and to enrage you. It will encourage you, we think, to learn that DMSO represents an exciting therapeutic principle, a therapeutic approach that for many disorders is safer and more effective than therapeutic approaches now in use, a therapeutic approach that offers new hope in diseases for which there is currently no known effective alternate treatment. And it will enrage you, we think, to discover that the real reason that DMSO is not yet a generally accepted therapeutic principle in medicine today in the United States has little to do with the safety or effectiveness of the substance but with considerations that place more value on regulatory procedures than on the right of individuals to live without pain or suffering.

Unfortunately, it is impossible to tell the true story of DMSO without calling into question many of the actions that the FDA, specifically the New Drug Section of the FDA, has taken with respect to DMSO over the past eighteen years. Exactly why the FDA has taken such an antagonistic position with respect to DMSO for so long is something neither of us has ever fully understood. In any event, as you read this book, please keep in mind that we are by no means against the idea of drug regulations *per se*. Obviously, there is need for a mechanism to insure that the drugs that people buy over the counter or through prescription are reasonably safe, properly prepared and useful. In the case of DMSO, however, we believe that the mechanism has failed to act in the best interests of the people of the United States. The question raised in the handling of DMSO by the FDA is whether bureaucrats should be involved in decisions concerning new drugs. And once you read this book and see for yourself the facts about DMSO, we think you'll agree.

ROBERT J. HERSCHLER
STANLEY W. JACOB

This book would not have been possible were it not for the help of a great many people, most of whom are mentioned in the text. Among those not mentioned who were instrumental in the book's development are Betsy Cenedella, Roger Cooper, Ned Kane, Kate Kelly, Elizabeth Frost Knappman, Kenneth Lane, Michael Remer, Nell Sutera and Loise Web.

Contents

CHAPTER I

===

In Search of a Panacea

Everybody knows there's no such thing as a panacea—a drug that can cure everything. And everybody knows that no drug is without side effects. But let's say, for the sake of argument, that somebody—the government, a drug company, a foundation—pulled together a blue-ribbon group of pharmacologists and physicians, presented them an unlimited budget and told them to develop a drug that came closer to being a panacea than any substance now known. Imagine the properties that such a drug, were it ever developed, would embody.

To begin with, the drug would be effective not only against one or two conditions and diseases, but against a broad range of maladies, from simple, everyday problems such as sprains and sinusitis to life-threatening diseases such as stroke or cancer. The drug, in other words, would be far more powerful than aspirin and a good deal more versatile than, say, penicillin.

Apart from its effectiveness, the drug would be safe,

keeping in mind that not even aspirin is completely harmless. Physicians who prescribed it wouldn't have to concern themselves with the adverse reactions that may claim as many as 30,000 to 60,000 lives a year in the United States alone. And the people who take it wouldn't have to suffer the myriad side effects—headache, fatigue, blurring of vision, mental disorientation—that come with the territory when you have a chronic disease for which there are only a handful of medications available.

The drug would also be versatile—versatile enough so that, depending on the condition, a physician could administer it orally or topically, by injection or intravenously. And it would be stable enough so that you could ship it anywhere in the world, or keep it on the shelf for months and not have to worry about it spoiling or losing its potency. The raw materials from which the drug was made would be readily available, so that you would never have to concern yourself with a shortage. And, finally, if you had a social conscience, you'd want the drug to be inexpensive enough (somewhat less expensive than, say, the interferon treatments now being offered for cancer in Europe at a price of $65,000) so that patients who took it on a long-term basis wouldn't have to spend a big chunk of their yearly income for the privilege of living without pain.

Well, as it happens, reports coming out of Portland, Oregon, during the mid-1960's suggested that a drug embodying all of these properties had indeed been discovered. Even the *New York Times*, in an editorial, described the drug as "the nearest thing to a wonder drug that the 1960's have produced so far."

The drug was remarkably versatile. It could bring quick and effective relief from ailments as varied as simple sprains and sinusitis to burns and arthritis. There was talk about its ability to stabilize progressively crippling arthritic conditions, and to alleviate certain forms of mental illness.

As far as anybody could tell, the drug also looked safe. People taking it were not suffering anywhere near the side effects that might be expected from similar doses of other, approved prescription drugs. Researchers were serving massive doses of it to laboratory animals, and finding it to have surprisingly little toxicity. What's more, the drug had a curious and remarkable property no other therapeutic substance was known to have: if you applied it to your skin, it managed somehow to get directly into your system without inflicting the damage associated with toxic chemicals—such as lye—endowed with the same penetrating capacity. You knew the drug was penetrating the skin because you could *taste* it within minutes after you applied it. It had a garlicky or, as some people described it, an oyster-like taste—not especially pleasant but not nauseatingly unpleasant, either. And the ability of the new drug to penetrate the skin without causing damage appeared to open up a new frontier of drug therapy: conceivably, you could mix it with other drugs that normally had to be given by injection, and the versatile new drug could carry these other drugs through the skin directly to the source of the problem.

Best of all, perhaps, this new substance was inexpensive and easily produced. It came from trees and was a bountiful by-product of the paper-making process. It could also be made from coal, petroleum or industrial wastes. Indeed, it was already on the market as an industrial solvent, and had been widely used for this purpose—particularly in the plastics industry—since the mid-1950's, because of its unusually good mixing properties; you could go into a chemical supply store and buy a pint of it—enough to last you at least a month—for about 35 cents.

The name of the new "wonder drug" was dimethyl sulfoxide—DMSO, for short. But it wasn't really a new chemical at all. It had originally been synthesized in 1866 by a Russian chemist named Alexander N. Saytzeff. In 1963, however, two men—a research chemist named Robert Herschler and a surgeon on the faculty of the University of Oregon Medical School named Dr. Stanley Jacob —were writing papers attributing to this chemical at least seven different and important medical properties, among them its ability to relieve pain, fight infection and reduce inflammation. Their clinical reports were promising enough and dramatic enough that many people, among them scientists, physicians and drug-industry executives, were calling DMSO the most important medical breakthrough since penicillin. And some people were going so far as to call DMSO the "aspirin of the twenty-first century."

That was in 1963. Today, in the early 1980's, there are still a great many people—more, in fact, than in 1963— who believe that DMSO is indeed a medical breakthrough that deserves to be called the "aspirin of the twenty-first century." Tens of thousands of people throughout the United States swear by its therapeutic benefits. Athletes —professional and amateur alike—have been using DMSO for years for sprains, pulls and other soft-tissue injuries, and one college trainer who has been conducting tests with DMSO over the past several years, Marv Robertson of Brigham Young University, states flatly that DMSO reduces the recovery time from soft-tissue injuries by "50 percent on the average" when compared to treatments now commonly used.

Besides this, DMSO is now being used regularly by thousands of arthritic patients, many of whom insist that it is the only effective pain-killer they have ever been able to take that spares them the fatigue, loss of appetite, anxiousness and irritability that other arthritis prescription drugs generally produce. People use DMSO for cuts, for sores, for itching conditions. Some people even rub it on their gums and will swear to you that if you do the same thing once every few weeks, your gums will never bleed when you brush your teeth. "I've used DMSO on serious cuts," says a Bozeman, Montana, man, "and they have always healed in less than half the time it used to take. I've used DMSO on a sprained ankle and saved a doctor bill and being off my feet for a week. I've used it for burns. For the physical well-being of my family, the worst blow that could come to us would be to find out we could no longer get DMSO." And Dr. Nat Wilson, a surgeon on the clinical faculty of the University of Oregon Health Sciences Center, goes so far as to say that if he had to choose only one drug to take with him to a desert island, he'd have trouble choosing between DMSO and aspirin.

It is also a fact that no therapeutic substance still unapproved for general use by the U.S. Food and Drug Administration has been the object of as many scientific studies as DMSO. Thousands of articles on DMSO have appeared in the world's scientific and medical literature since 1964, and the implications behind many of these articles are startling. Several reports offer convincing evidence in animal studies that DMSO could save lives, help to reduce—and in some cases actually *prevent*—the paralytic effects of severe head and spinal cord injuries. Some suggest that DMSO, together with other substances, could help accelerate the physical, social and intellectual development of mentally retarded children. And some studies—including one written by one of the world's most prominent cancer researchers, Charlotte Friend, of the Center for Experimental Cell Biology at Mount Sinai School of Medicine, in New York—suggest that DMSO is destined to play an important role in the search for an ultimate understanding of cancer.

That's one side of the DMSO picture. The other side of the picture is that, as of the summer of 1981—nearly nineteen years after the discovery of its medical benefits—

DMSO is an "approved" drug in the United States for only one condition, a rare and painful bladder disease known as interstitial cystitis. Part of this same side of the picture is the official position of the FDA, which is that DMSO remains an "unproven drug," never mind its being prescribed in one form or another in Canada, and in Switzerland, Great Britain, Germany and dozens of other countries throughout Europe and South America. And part of this side of the picture is that as many as a million Americans are buying DMSO that has been manufactured for commercial use but using it on themselves for medical purposes, most of them unsure of how pure the commercial grade is, or even how to best use the substance.

The result is a debate of escalating proportions. On one side stands a group of physicians, scientists and a zealous army of patients who maintain that DMSO works, is safe and ought to be approved as soon as possible so that the public can reap its benefits. (Some people who take this position argue that DMSO should become available with or without FDA approval, so that the public doesn't have to risk the black-market substance.) On the other side stands a government agency, together with certain segments of the medical establishment, insisting that the verdict on DMSO is still out—that its safety and effectiveness have not yet been proven, and that until such time that proof is demonstrated in "scientifically valid" studies, the drug must be considered medically unproven and potentially dangerous.

The debate is not new. It has been going on, in fact, since 1965, when the FDA ordered a halt to all clinical tests on humans that were being done by six different drug companies seeking FDA approval for DMSO medications. As the reason for its suspension of testing, the FDA cited laboratory reports which showed that some animals given very high dosages of DMSO developed changes in the lenses of their eyes. But there is evidence to suggest that FDA officials simply used these test reports as a pretext to ease the pressure that the public and elected officials were putting on the federal agency to give the drug its approval. Typically, when a new drug is being tested for safety and effectiveness before being approved by the FDA, the public has no way of getting hold of the substance; but because DMSO was obtainable as a commercial solvent, the FDA had no means of controlling its medicinal uses. "Two weeks after the FDA halted studies," Dr. Stanley Jacob told Senator Edward M. Kennedy at a Senate Health Subcommittee hearing on July 31, 1980, "they called inspectors from the major districts in the United States to Washington and they said, in essence, 'we are not sure of ourselves; this is probably a safe drug and it is probably an effective drug; go out and justify what we did and find us some pigeons.' Following that," continued Jacob, "they launched into the most vigorous investigation that had ever been done by the FDA up to that point. It was so vigorous that they had to call in the FBI because there were some 1,500 physician investigators in the United States studying the merit of the new drug."

But regardless of the FDA's motives, its actions with respect to DMSO went largely unnoticed by the public until a Sunday evening in March, 1980, when the CBS news magazine program *60 Minutes* presented a segment on DMSO that generated more viewer response than any other segment *60 Minutes* had ever run. It prompted such an avalanche of phone calls to the University of Oregon Health Sciences Center, the headquarters of Dr. Stanley Jacob's DMSO clinic, that the university had to hire eight additional telephone operators for several weeks. It sent thousands of Americans scurrying to their veterinarians (DMSO is an approved drug for veterinary uses) and their chemical supply stores. And it created, overnight, a new industry: underground DMSO. Although you couldn't get DMSO legally from a doctor or pharmacy, you could buy it on road stands in Arizona, on Indian reservations in the state of Washington, and in health food stores across the country, just as long as everyone understood that you were buying DMSO as a *solvent* and not as a medicine. Ads began to appear in newspapers throughout the country. Not only could you write in or call a toll-free number to have some "solvent" DMSO sent to you, you could also inquire about setting up your own DMSO *franchise*. The profit margin was an entrepreneur's fantasy. The same DMSO you could buy in its commercial-grade form for sixty cents a pint could be sold on the underground DMSO market for about twenty dollars a pint—tax free.

In the wake of this new surge of interest triggered by the *60 Minutes* broadcast, a flood of newspaper and magazine articles have appeared, generating even more interest in and more debate about DMSO. Most of the articles have presented a fairly balanced picture, but the FDA has felt duty-bound to reiterate its position, warning the public that DMSO is *not* an approved drug for medical purposes other than interstitial cystitis, that its effectiveness has *not* yet been established and that its safety can *not* be guaranteed. The DMSO being peddled on the underground market, moreover, could well have toxic impurities. All of which serves to confuse an already perplexed American public all the more.

"The story of DMSO is a sad story," said a somber Edward M. Kennedy in his opening remarks at a Senate Subcommittee hearing on DMSO held on July 31, 1980—one of a number of federal and state hearings that have been held on DMSO as the controversy has continued to boil. "It is sad," Kennedy explained, "because hundreds of thousands of Americans suffering from a variety of painful and often disabling diseases have placed their hopes in this drug, and yet, after eighteen years, we still do not know whether or not those hopes are misplaced."

Kennedy went on to depict the DMSO story as a story

of "failure." He criticized the FDA for its failure to "handle the drug appropriately." He criticized the private sector for not adequately monitoring the quality of the scientific work that has been done on DMSO. "This failure of both government and industrial responsibility has had a very high cost," he said. "The erosion of public confidence in the ability of government—in this case, the FDA—to work, to respond to human suffering, to meet people's need."

A very high cost indeed, not only in the "erosion of public confidence," but in the suffering that millions of Americans have endured because of the manner in which the issue has been handled over the past fifteen years.

For there is no question but that DMSO is a compound with properties unlike any other compound known to mankind; its membrane-penetrating properties alone make it a substance with a vast range of medical potential. And there remains little argument that when properly administered, DMSO is probably as safe a pharmaceutical substance, safer even, than aspirin—almost certainly an excellent and safe therapy for most soft-tissue injuries, and probably better than any therapy now available.

There is also convincing clinical and laboratory evidence to suggest that DMSO, either by itself or as an adjunct with other drugs, offers hope to many of the more than 31 million Americans who suffer from the various forms of arthritis but have yet to find a drug or treatment modality that reduces their pain and inflammation without causing disabling side effects.

Clinical reports out of the DMSO Clinic in Portland, Oregon, show that even rheumatoid arthritis patients, if treated properly with DMSO, experience pain relief and increased mobility and—perhaps more importantly—respond in a way that suggests their condition is stabilizing as the result of DMSO treatment. Recent studies reported from Russia and Japan, where DMSO figures prominently in arthritis research, show that, by triggering the excretion of certain immunity-related factors believed to be causal agents in rheumatoid arthritis symptoms, it may well be able to *stabilize* what has long been considered the progressive pattern of crippling effects of this disease. Other studies suggest that DMSO protects the "lubricating" material in the affected joint from losing its lubricity.

Possibly more dramatic is the potential for using DMSO to treat a number of diseases for which no other effective or low-risk treatment exists. There is evidence from South America, for instance—evidence gathered by experienced physicians and specialists—that DMSO, together with certain neurotransmitters, can help children afflicted with the mental retardation condition known as Down's syndrome to become more responsive to their environment. In many cases, this enhanced responsiveness can mean the difference between a virtually helpless child and one that can dress itself, control its bowels and bladder, and perform simple household tasks. DMSO appears to be measurably helpful to paraplegics and quadriplegics. Many paralytic patients currently using DMSO report prompt relief of many of the symptoms usually associated with paraplegia and quadriplegia: less pain, fewer bedsores and bladder infections and less fatigue than before. Furthermore, several of these patients show signs of actually regaining certain functions that quadriplegics and paraplegics, according to conventional thinking, are not supposed to recover. And a series of studies, the bulk of them done by Dr. Jack de la Torre, a physician and Ph.D. formerly of the University of Chicago School of Medicine and now based at the University of Miami, show that if administered soon enough, DMSO can save the lives and prevent paralysis of laboratory animals that have been subjected to normally fatal or paralyzing head and spinal-cord injuries, as well as to the kind of brain damage that generally occurs in strokes. Limited human studies now underway confirm the ability of DMSO to stabilize some of the conditions that lead to death or paralysis in human head and spinal-cord injury victims. So it is not outrageous to speculate that if DMSO had been in hospital and emergency rooms or in ambulances over the past fifteen years, a substantial proportion of the victims of head and spinal-cord injuries would be living reasonably normal lives today instead of being confined to wheelchairs, unable to control life processes as basic as bladder function.

These are big statements, admittedly, and it would be reckless to make them if there weren't solid evidence to back them up. Nobody appreciates this fact more than the two men who have been in the eye of the DMSO storm from the beginning, Robert Herschler and Stanley Jacob. For nearly twenty years, Herschler, the chemist, and Jacob, the physician, have, at their own financial expense, and at the expense of their personal careers, led the crusade for the approval of DMSO. Robert Herschler lost his research job because of his refusal to adhere to his company's directives that he take no public stand in the DMSO controversy. Stanley Jacob has been vilified time and again by many of his colleagues in the medical profession for being "unprofessional" in his statements and actions throughout the controversy. "I don't know what 'unprofessional' means," says Jacob, who spends an average of 70 to 80 hours a week working at the University of Oregon Health Sciences Center. "I'm a physician. My role in life is to do what I can to relieve people of their sickness, pain and suffering. How can I keep silent when I know without any question that millions of Americans are suffering needlessly because of a government agency position that isn't based on science but on politics."

Unless you have actually been to the DMSO Clinic in Portland, have spoken to nurses and patients, have read case reports, scientific studies and FDA correspondence, and have spent time with Jacob and Herschler themselves, you are probably justified in being somewhat skeptical of their motives in this entire affair. It has been suggested, for instance, that Robert Herschler and Stanley Jacob are much more interested in promoting DMSO for their personal gain than they are in advancing the cause of medical science. And if you watched a Mike Douglas show in early 1981, you might have heard author-surgeon Dr. William Nolen observe that Robert Herschler stood to become a millionaire many times over when—and if—DMSO gets FDA approval.

But the facts speak otherwise. True, as discoverers of the medical properties of DMSO, Herschler and Jacob are entitled to a percentage of royalties from DMSO sales until the patents run out in the mid- to late 1980's. But neither man has reaped any financial benefit to date from DMSO, and both men have turned down lucrative business offers that could have made them extremely wealthy within a matter of months. Whatever royalties the two have received have been put back into DMSO research, the records of which can be verified in the public domain. Under modified patent agreements now in effect, Jacob signs over all the proceeds he may derive from the royalties resulting from DMSO drug sales to the University of Oregon Health Sciences Center Foundation, and Herschler signs over his share of the proceeds to the newly formed DMSO Research Institute.

"If money were our motivation," Jacob says, "Bob and I could have attached our names to a DMSO clinic in Mexico and probably grossed more than $30 million a year, but money isn't now, nor has ever been our motivation."

Not that we're dealing here with a pair of saints. Both men admit that they've been guilty of poor judgment at various stages of the DMSO controversy, and neither man is blind to his own or to each other's weaknesses. Indeed, as close as Jacob and Herschler are today, there was a period during the late 1960's when they rarely spoke to one another. Jacob, who is more gregarious than Herschler but also more impulsive, has time and again gotten himself into difficulty because he is oblivious to bureaucratic procedures and finds it next to impossible to say no to anybody who seeks a favor or asks for his help. And Herschler, who is as disdainful of bureaucracy as Jacob, has shown little restraint in his public statements about the FDA, not to mention his former employer, the Crown Zellerbach Corporation. "I suppose if I worked at it," Herschler says, "I could learn to express my feelings a little more diplomatically, but it's probably too late in the game to change."

It ought to be pointed out, too, that neither Jacob nor Herschler is anti-FDA to the degree that they don't recognize the need for some mechanism by which the safety of drugs that reach the marketplace can be guaranteed. "It isn't so much the FDA itself that has created the problem we're now facing," says Herschler, "as much as it is a group of individuals in one department—the new drug evaluation section." Herschler grants to this agency their right and duty to make sure that drugs are safe and effective, but questions the actions of the department since 1965 with respect to DMSO and against the physicians and investigators involved with DMSO. "I don't think the FDA," he says, "has the right to pressure physicians so much that they're afraid to prescribe the drug. I don't think they have the right to interfere with the doctor–patient relationship, which, in the final analysis, is what they've been doing for the past sixteen years with DMSO."

But personalities and politics apart, the real question here has to do with DMSO itself. What is it? How effective is it? Is it safe? What conditions does it help relieve? What have laboratory and clinical studies shown about its medical potential?

This book will attempt to answer these and other questions about DMSO. The purpose of the book is not to encourage you to use DMSO on your own or to show you how to administer it. As we have said and as you will see in reading this book, DMSO is unlike other drugs. It is more a therapeutic principle than a drug in the pure sense of the term, and its medical benefits are as much a function of *how* it is administered as they are of how much of it is administered. As with anything you take to treat any problem, you should always check with your doctor before using DMSO on yourself. Many doctors in the past have been reluctant to recommend DMSO to their patients, but as the clinical evidence on DMSO's effectiveness mounts, more and more doctors are learning how to work with it and recommending it over standard therapy in many situations.

"Twenty-five years from now," says Stanley Jacob, "we're going to look back on what's happened with DMSO, and people are going to wonder why it took us so long to take advantage of its medical benefits. Maybe by then, when the *next* DMSO comes along, it won't take twenty years to provide its benefits to the public."

CHAPTER II

The Discovery

There would be no DMSO controversy today if in the late 1950's, the Crown Zellerbach Corporation, one of the world's largest paper-processing concerns, had not asked a young research chemist at its Camas, Washington, chemical products division to find some new commercial possibilities for one of the by-products of its wood pulp manufacturing operation—dimethyl sulfoxide. The chemist, Robert Herschler, had grown up in Oregon and graduated from Washington University, in St. Louis. He was thirty-five, a tall, good-looking but reticent man who was more comfortable in a laboratory or off by himself fly fishing than he was at social gatherings. He was married, had three daughters and lived in a house he had designed and built himself.

Herschler describes himself today as a "competent but not brilliant" chemist. He has always been a creative problem-solver and an alert observer, and one of the first things he observed about DMSO, as he was probing for agricultural uses for the substance, was that when he mixed it with certain plant and tree antibiotics and fungicidal agents, the agents penetrated more deeply and more quickly into the circulatory system of the plants and trees than the antibiotics and fungicides did on their own. DMSO, in other words, seemed to have a very strong "carrier effect."

Herschler also noticed—couldn't help it, really—that whenever he inadvertently got DMSO on his hands, he would quickly develop a funny, oyster-like taste in his mouth. Other investigators had undoubtedly experienced the same thing, but probably assumed the taste arose from the vapor. Herschler had a different view. He suspected the DMSO was penetrating the skin and getting directly into his system.

As a chemist, Herschler knew that any number of chemical substances have this same power. Ammonia, for instance, can penetrate biological membranes, even the skin. So can gasoline, naphtha and many of the chemicals found in pesticides. The difference, though, is that compounds like ammonia, before breaching the skin barrier, first destroy the integrity of the barrier. As far as Herschler could tell, DMSO, apart from a slight burning sensation when it first came into contact with the skin, wasn't doing much harm at all. Outside of the funny taste, Herschler couldn't see that the substance was producing any of the reactions —nausea, headache, sweating or anything else—that a toxic substance might be expected to produce once it got into the system.

Herschler soon discovered other properties of this curious substance. One evening, while working in the small laboratory he had built in his Camas, Washington, home, he accidentally spilled some mustard-gas-like poison on his hand and arm. Blisters erupted. The skin became inflamed. "I reached for the DMSO," Herschler remembers, "because I knew it could draw water away from the blisters. What astonished me was that the pain disappeared within minutes, and so did the blisters."

Herschler immediately told his superiors at Crown Zellerbach what he was finding out about DMSO, but his superiors demonstrated no excitement about the chemical's medicinal possibilities. (The company, remember, was in the lumber and paper business and not in the drug business.) "They just didn't share my fascination with DMSO and they weren't about to give me any money to support further research," Herschler says. "After a while I stopped beating my head against the wall. I figured if I had discovered something important, I was going to need a better facility to test out some hypotheses. I was desperate to find someone who could test DMSO in a clinical environment."

Enter Stanley Jacob. At thirty-seven, Jacob was the same age as Herschler when the two men met, but, unlike the chemist, had been raised in the East and Midwest. In high school Jacob had been a cheerleader, a Ping-Pong whiz, a state debating champion and the president of his senior class. A science major at Ohio State University who graduated at the top of his class, he received his M.D. from Ohio State three years later. He took his surgical training in the Harvard system, and was appointed an instructor in surgery at Harvard Medical School. Since 1959 Jacob had been assistant professor of surgery at the University of Oregon Health Sciences Center and when he met Herschler was in the second year of a five-year Markle Scholarship in the Medical Sciences, one of the highest awards the medical profession bestows on its young practitioners.

Jacob had his own reasons for being interested in DMSO. His research specialty was cryobiology—a science that involves freezing and preserving surgically removed organs for future transplantation. Looking for ways to protect organs from the damage they usually undergo during freezing, Jacob was intrigued by a study published in

England during the late 1950's indicating that DMSO was an effective preservation agent. But once he and Herschler got together and Herschler began sharing with Jacob his observations, experiences and thoughts concerning the chemical, Jacob's interest in DMSO caught fire—and for reasons that had nothing to do with cryobiology. "The stuff fascinated me right from the start," Jacob now says. "I had a gut feeling, just as Bob did, that we were on to something very big and very important."

With frequent input from Herschler, Jacob began experimenting with DMSO on his laboratory animals. At this early stage, he points out, their interest was focused on the drug's carrier properties. If DMSO could penetrate the skin without causing irreversible damage, he and Herschler wondered, could it not then carry substances that normally had to be administered by injection? And could it not then go a long way to solve one of the ongoing problems in drug therapy—the fact that many drugs, when taken orally, lose much of their potency in the gastrointestinal tract before they've had a chance to do their job in the body? Both men wondered—incorrectly, as it turned out—whether diabetics might be able to take their daily insulin by mixing it with DMSO and rubbing it onto their skin. And both were excited over the possibility that DMSO, by taking certain substances past the blood-brain barrier, the body's built-in protection system that prevents all but a few substances from passing from the blood into the brain and spinal cord, could represent a breakthrough in the pharmacological treatment of mental illness.

What concerned both Herschler and Jacob, however, was whether a drug as powerful and seemingly effective as DMSO could also be safe. Subsequently, most of the early experiments with DMSO were designed to see how much of the drug you had to give to laboratory animals before they died or got sick. Jacob flooded his laboratory animals with DMSO. Using concentrations of 80 percent or higher of the substance, he overdosed rats topically (on the skin), rectally, intravenously and even orally. To his surprise, he found that even in very high dosages, DMSO had a relatively low level of toxicity.

Comfortable in the knowledge that DMSO was safe, Jacob began using it on himself—something Herschler and his friends had already been doing for years. He also tested it on some of his co-workers who were now getting caught up in his excitement. He confirmed Herschler's findings that if you put DMSO on a sprained ankle, the pain and swelling would subside almost immediately, and he found that DMSO could cure cold sores on the lips of the nurses at the hospital and that it could cut the pain and significantly lessen the scarring of burns. Putting some DMSO on the forehead of a Portland State College football player, Jacob found that it cleared the player's headache within minutes. And he remembers in particular that one morning while accompanying an intern through the Health Sciences Center hospital, he applied some DMSO to a six-year-old girl who had been suffering for most of her life with rheumatoid arthritis and hadn't known a pain-free day for the past three years. "A half hour after I'd rubbed the DMSO on her shoulder and neck, she turned her head and moved her shoulder," Jacob recalls. "She hadn't done that for two years. Then I lifted her out of the crib and coaxed her to walk with the intern and me helping her. She took a few steps and started to cry. When we asked her why she was crying, she said: 'Because it doesn't hurt anymore.'"

Now both Jacob and Herschler were well-schooled scientists, and didn't need to be reminded that a case for a new medical discovery isn't built on the basis of a handful of animal experiments and some isolated clinical incidents. Yet both men were keen observers, and the more they observed, the more convinced they became that they had stumbled across a truly remarkable substance. "We were finding out new things about DMSO every day," Herschler remembers. "We knew that the experiments we were doing weren't the most elaborately controlled. Then again, we were working on a shoestring, and we were dealing with a very unpredictable substance. We kept reminding ourselves that we had to stay objective. But we were seeing things that made objectivity very difficult." The substance that was so much a source of fascination to Robert Herschler and Stanley Jacob in the early 1960's and remains to this day so much a source of fascination to both men looks, at first glance, like ordinary drinking water. But the resemblance ends right there, and the mystery of its properties to so many of the users of DMSO is all right with Herschler and Jacob who admit that much of what DMSO can do is a mystery to them as well.

The big problem in trying to understand DMSO is that it is noticeably and confoundingly idiosyncratic in the way in which it interacts with various tissues and organs in the body. In some instances—its effects on the kidneys, for example—DMSO *stimulates* function. In other instances—such as its effect on certain nerve fibers believed to be centrally involved in pain—it *inhibits* function, which is to say, limits pain. Furthermore, DMSO seems to work better in certain individuals than in others, but for reasons that nobody knows. Indeed DMSO can affect the same individual differently on different occasions. "It's fickle stuff," says Oregon marathon runner Albert Salazar, "sometimes I get immediate relief, and other times it doesn't seem to work at all on a similar problem. It's mysterious."

Contributing to the mystery of DMSO is the fact that it does a lot of things that conventional medical and scientific wisdom have long held aren't supposed to be done by a chemical substance. For one thing, says Robert Herschler, "Prior to our studies with DMSO during the early 1960's it was an accepted medical principle that drug vehicles (like DMSO) could only penetrate membranes, including the skin, by first causing irreversible damage. Most scientists wouldn't believe that DMSO passed safely across membranes until they tried it themselves."

Exactly how DMSO can move in and out of membranes without causing irreversible changes in the structure of these membranes isn't fully understood. Then again, nobody is absolutely sure of how membranes themselves can be so selective about which substances they allow into cells and which substances they repel. Herschler's guess is that DMSO is so similar to water in its basic biochemical actions that the body, for all intents and purposes, doesn't differentiate the two substances: everywhere water goes in the body, DMSO will also go—even past the so-called blood-brain barrier, whose function it is to keep all but essential substances from the brain. "DMSO never functions *alone* in the body," says Herschler, "but always in concert with water. The two substances are drawn to each other, and they mix very well. Whenever DMSO is present in any tissues, water will be there as well."

Like water, DMSO is a superior solvent—a substance capable of dissolving other materials. In fact, years before its medical properties were first discovered, DMSO was widely used in the plastics industry and in the manufacture of synthetic fibers. It has the power to liquefy many of the materials from which fiber mills fashion synthetic threads, and it is a superior medium for special chemical reactions. (Despite the fact that black-market DMSO is sold as a "degreaser," it's actually an ineffective solvent for cutting grease.) Yet DMSO, like water, once it gets inside the body, operates in a beneficial way. It supports many of the same basic, life-sustaining chemical reactions that water supports, and like water it acts as an insulator, preventing adverse reactions from taking place. But DMSO is sufficiently different from water in its biochemical makeup as to trigger certain interactions that water itself can't trigger. "Other solvents have some of the same biochemical capabilities as DMSO," says Herschler, "but they don't move as freely through the body as DMSO. They can't move in and out of membranes. What's unique about DMSO is that it does a lot of things in the body that various substances are capable of doing, but does these things at sites other substances can't get to, and does them in a safe way."

The fact that DMSO could penetrate the skin and could move freely in and out of other membranes throughout the body represented to Herschler and Jacob a new frontier of treatment.

"Bob and I started talking in terms of something Bob called 'focus therapy,'" says Jacob. "We were fascinated by the idea of being able to take a substance that you'd normally have to administer either orally or by a needle, mix it with DMSO and then apply it right to the site of the injury. When you do this, you can reduce the amount of the substance you'd normally give orally. This means cutting down on side effects, and enabling a patient to take a drug for longer periods of time without developing a tolerance for it. It was a revolutionary idea at the time."

Another thing that excited both men about DMSO was that it could do so many of the things other prescription drugs could do—such as reduce pain and inflammation, relax muscles and increase blood flow to injured areas— without serious side effects. Says Herschler: "Pharmacologists took for granted at the time—and still do today —that any drug with the capacity of doing good has to cause a lot of side effects, but we weren't seeing any side effects with DMSO except for the taste, the odor and a mild rash that some people got at the site of application."

Yet another thing about DMSO that made it so unusual was that no substance with all of its medicinal properties was so abundant or easily produced. Herschler points out that nature herself produces DMSO. "One of DMSO's main metabolites—dimethyl sulfide—can be found in abundance in virtually all marine plant life," he points out. "In tropical climates the sun draws dimethyl sulfide into the atmosphere where it reacts in the ozone layer to form DMSO." The result: the presence of trace amounts of DMSO in all rainfall of marine origin. As Herschler likes to put it, "DMSO is probably the only therapeutic compound that mother nature herself likes to make above cloud level."

Finally, DMSO differs from other medications in that its action against a disease process doesn't weaken with time. Most patients using DMSO for long periods find, in fact, that they can use less with continued benefit.

The DMSO produced in the United States is largely a by-product of the process in which wood pulp is made into paper; other countries use industrial waste products or by-products of coal or petroleum as the basic materials for their DMSO manufacture. "The fact that you could make DMSO so inexpensively struck Stanley and me from the beginning as one of its valuable features," says Herschler. "Here was a drug that could be manufactured so cheaply that anybody in the world could afford to use it. What we didn't count on is that FDA regulations would increase the cost from sixty cents a pound to fifteen dollars, for the approved DMSO. If plain ocean water was found to have drug value, and had to go through the FDA approval process, it would end up costing ten dollars an ounce!"

The Basic Properties of DMSO

Most drugs embody at most one or two basic pharmacological properties. Some drugs relieve pain. Some stimulate the heart. Some suppress the action of certain organs, relax muscles, fight infection, help the body get rid of water, help the body retain water—and so forth. DMSO does a lot of different things. Many drugs can outperform DMSO in one specific area—drugs that are more powerful in their antibacterial effect, drugs that are more rapid acting anti-inflammatory agents, drugs that relax muscles more quickly. But no substance known does as many things as DMSO does without producing serious side effects. Here is a brief summary of DMSO's principal properties.

Getting Past the Membrane

More than any other feature, it is the ability of DMSO to penetrate biological membranes without permanently altering or damaging the membrane structure that makes it so pharmacologically interesting. Ammonia, gasoline and naphtha will all penetrate membranes, but in doing so, bulldoze their way through. In contrast, says Herschler, "imagine a dune buggy on a beach. The buggy moves by conforming to the shape of the dunes. That's how DMSO tends to operate." Rather than bulldozing its way through skin like a drill, he explains, "it slips in and out of tiny membrane spaces."

One theory for the way in which DMSO manages to move safely through membranes, suggested in the *Annual Review of Pharmacology* in 1972, is that certain insoluble substances in tissue water are bonded together and wrapped in an "ice-like sheath" of water. The water molecules in this sheath have the ability either to "accept" or to "donate" hydrogen atoms and become attached—through these hydrogen atoms—to proteins, forming so-called "hydrogen bonds." Enter DMSO, which is a hydrogen bond *acceptor*. It replaces the water molecule that is "bound" to the proteins and interacts with these proteins in a way that temporarily changes the geometric shape of the protein molecule. The change lets DMSO penetrate the sheath and pass through the membrane. When water once again takes the place of the DMSO in the sheath, the protein configuration resumes its original form.

Another theory is that DMSO penetrates membranes through an osmotic effect—building up a pressure on the exterior of the membrane and changing the chemical conformation of the membrane in ways that allow DMSO to move in and out. As soon as DMSO leaves, the membrane returns to its original state.

Whatever the mechanism, one thing is clear. The penetrating power of DMSO varies from membrane to membrane. It varies, too, according to the concentration of DMSO: that is, how much pure DMSO is in the solution with respect to water.

DMSO solutions of 50 percent or less, for instance, do not move through the skin at as rapid a rate as higher percentages of DMSO do. This explains why patients seeking pain relief from the only prescriptive DMSO— the 50 percent Rimso solution—are generally disappointed.

The lesser concentrations simply don't build up enough osmotic pressure to penetrate the skin. Solutions as weak as 15 percent will penetrate membranes such as the urinary bladder wall.

DMSO as a Pain Reliever

When you apply it to the skin, DMSO will cut pain better than any other topical substance commonly used in medicine today. It is especially effective in reducing the pain of acute injuries, such as sprains, burns and cuts. Relief usually comes quickly (in burns, you can feel the effect in a moment or two) and will usually last from four to six hours. For DMSO to be effective as a topical analgesic, it must usually constitute at least 70 percent of a solution in which the other 30 percent is water. Lesser concentrations don't penetrate the skin barrier quickly enough to produce noticeable relief.

"In our clinical experience," says Stanley Jacob, "the *more* DMSO you use and the broader the area you cover, the more effectively it relieves pain. In an acute pain situation, like a bad sprain or a burn, we'll apply DMSO as frequently as every two or three hours."

DMSO is also an effective pain reliever for various types of chronic pain, but its analgesic effects in these chronic conditions are not as dramatic as in acute states. In some cases, it may be six weeks or more before a patient with a chronic pain problem begins to experience noticeable pain relief from DMSO. In most instances, though, these are patients for whom no other safe, long-term pain-killer has worked. Chronic pain patients who do not respond to topical DMSO treatment are often helped with injections of a lower concentration of DMSO.

The mechanism by which DMSO reduces pain is not fully understood (then again, pain itself is not a clearly understood phenomenon). Many researchers relate it to DMSO's ability to slow down and, in some cases, entirely halt the conduction of pain signals from the brain to the injured site through certain nerve fibers thought to be implicated in the transmission of pain signals. Animal studies confirm that DMSO's moderating effect on nerve fiber activity is *transitory*. Once the DMSO leaves the system, the nerve activity resumes its normal activity.

DMSO's pain-reducing capacity has been established in dozens of clinical and laboratory studies. (See chapter IV.) A study conducted in 1980 by two pharmacologists— H. J. Haigler and D. D. Spring—at Emory University in Atlanta shows that DMSO can be as effective a pain-killer in experimental rats as the narcotic morphine, producing pain relief for a longer period of time and without the danger of addiction.

DMSO as an Antibacterial Agent

Although DMSO has mild antibacterial properties of its own, its most important antibacterial action appears to be its ability to reduce the resistance of bacteria that have become insensitive to certain antibiotic drugs. Many bacteria develop resistance to certain antibiotics through changes in the outer membrane of the bacterial cell. In 1966, G. E. Pottz and his colleagues (*DMSO Symposium, Vienna*, 1966, G. Laudahn and K. Gertich, eds.) showed that when pretreated with 5 percent DMSO, the bacterial organism that causes tuberculosis became almost 200 times more sensitive to streptomycin a widely used antibiotic. Similar sensitizing effects have been found with many of the organisms that produce infections in the body: dose them with DMSO and they lose their capacity to resist attack by an antibiotic drug.

Suggests Jacob: "Rather than spend hundreds of millions of dollars over the next fifty years developing antibiotics that can overcome the problem of bacterial insensitivity, let's work with what we have, using DMSO as the sensitizing agent together with the antibiotics already proven as safe and effective." Russian scientists have already demonstrated this in man.

DMSO as an Anti-inflammatory Agent

Inflammation, best described as a tissue's reaction to injury, can occur because of a trauma—a sprain, cut, burn or other damage—secondary to an illness, following heat or cold or because of microorganisms. DMSO reduces inflammation in a number of different ways. For one thing, it has the ability to remove free radicals from an injury site (the concentration of free radicals invariably increases whenever there is inflammation). DMSO also has the ability to stabilize membranes, permitting the membrane to slow or stop any leakage of cell material from injured cells. Besides these properties, DMSO has also been shown (D. L. Berliner and G. G. Ruhman, "The Influence of DMSO on Fibroblastic Proliferation," *Ann. New York Academy of Science,* 141, 638, 1967) to inhibit the spread of fibroblasts.

Furthermore, although not as potent as cortisone in its anti-inflammatory properties, DMSO has fewer side effects. It can also be used in conjuction with other anti-inflammatory agents (including cortisone), allowing a physician to reduce the dosage of these agents and, in this manner, cut down on side effects.

DMSO as a Collagen-Softening Agent

Collagen is a protein normally found in many tissues throughout the body, particularly in connective tissue, such as that in the tendons; the collagen in animals gives us the food gelatin. But collagen is a culprit in a broad range of so-called collagen diseases, among them arthritis, hardening of the arteries and rheumatic fever in which accumulations of collagen interfere with normal function. While only one or two studies to date have shown that DMSO can *remove* abnormal levels of collagen in the body, there is considerable clinical evidence to indicate that DMSO can *soften* collagen and bring symptomatic relief to people suffering from diseases in which collagen interferes with basic life functions.

DMSO as a Diuretic

The body's ability to rid itself of water it doesn't need and, in the process, rid itself of acids, waste products and toxic substances through the urine is one of the basic processes of life. DMSO is one of a number of substances that enhance the flow and the volume of urine. Applied topically, DMSO has a very mild diuretic—or water eliminating—effect, but when given intravenously, it becomes one of the most powerful diuretics known. Rapid diuresis takes on special importance in certain types of injuries—serious head and spinal cord for instance—in which an excess amount of tissue fluid, known as edema, builds up and threatens areas that control critical functions. Clinical reports from the University of Oregon Health Sciences Center show that in emergency situations, DMSO can induce the body to excrete roughly three quarts of urine within an hour. These reports are backed up by laboratory studies showing that DMSO can increase the output of urine to ten times the normal level (K. Formaneck and R. Suckert, "Diuretische Wirkung von DMSO," in *DMSO Symposium, Vienna,* 1966, G. Laudahn and K. Gertich, eds., Saladruck, Berlin). DMSO increases urine output in two ways: first, by exerting a gentle osmotic pressure on the kidney cells that produce urine; and, second, by altering the flow of fluids through the membranes of the kidney filtration system.

DMSO as a Cholinesterase Inhibitor

Cholinesterase is an enzyme whose chief function in the body is to control the amount of another chemical—acetylcholine—that accumulates in nerve cells. Before a muscle can move, acetylcholine must reach a level that will enable the nerve fiber controlling the muscle to trigger the impulse that stimulates the muscle to move.

DMSO's potential to moderate the acetylcholine action through its inhibitory effect on cholinesterase might help explain the small but measureable increases in muscle activity that some paraplegics and quadriplegics experience after receiving DMSO treatment for several months. It may also offer a theoretical explanation for the improvement that some retarded children show after being on DMSO treatment for several months. "It's not a *dramatic* effect," says Stanley Jacob. "But it's very possible that over an extended period, the increased acetylcholine activity brings about a gradual improvement in the transmission of impulses in the nervous system."

DMSO as a Vasodilator

When the blood vessels constrict, the blood flow into affected areas of the body is reduced. When the blood vessels dilate, or widen, the blood flow increases. Following its application to the skin, DMSO's ability to dilate blood vessels is connected, at least in part, to the release of a substance known as histamine. The vasodilating properties of DMSO help account for its ability to bring rapid relief to sprains (i.e., it increases the flow of oxygen and other nutrients to the injured area) and partially account for its therapeutic benefits in the treatment of severe head and spinal-cord injuries.

DMSO as a Carrier of Other Drugs

Hundreds of animal studies have confirmed DMSO's ability to carry with it, across membranes, substances that wouldn't normally penetrate membranes on their own, but these studies also show that DMSO is a highly selective carrier. Substances of a lower molecular weight penetrate membranes more readily when mixed with DMSO than do substances of a high molecular weight; however, the shape of a molecule and its electrochemical makeup are also factors in its penetrating ability. Penicillin, steroids and cortisone are among the many medications whose penetrating powers are enhanced by mixing with DMSO. Insulin, however, *doesn't* pass through the skin when mixed with DMSO. DMSO's carrier potential is directly proportional to the strength of the solution, although for some curious reason 90 percent DMSO solution is a better transporter for some substances than 100 percent DMSO solution.

Some people speculate that DMSO's carrier potential raises the danger of toxic substances getting into the system, but Robert Herschler says the danger is exaggerated. "Although there are some toxic substances found in pesticides and insect sprays that DMSO could conceivably take into the body," he says, "the only way you're in any danger is if moments after you put DMSO on you walk outside and get directly into the path of somebody spraying some trees. Even then, you'd have plenty of time to wash it off before you'd experience any adverse effects."

DMSO as a Reducer or Enhancer of Drug Action

Apart from its ability to carry certain substances across the skin barrier, DMSO interacts with various drugs in a variety of ways. Yet there doesn't appear to be a pattern that would allow researchers to predict whether DMSO will enhance or reduce the activity of any special drug or drug class.

DMSO's interaction with many commonly prescribed drugs shows a conflicting pattern. When DMSO is combined with digitoxin, a compound similar to the commonly prescribed heart medication digitalis, the effects of digitoxin are enhanced. When certain drugs used routinely in the treatment of mental illness—chlorpromazine, for instance—are administered with DMSO, no enhancing effects occur. DMSO's effects on the body when mixed with alcohol vary enormously, depending on the dosage of each and how the DMSO is administered. "There's no way you can predict the effects that combinations of drugs are going to have on individual patients," says Stanley Jacob. "It's a highly individual phenomenon, and the more conservative one is the better. We're beginning to understand how DMSO interacts with certain *types* of drugs," he explains, "but this particular branch of pharmacology is such a new field it's going to be a long time before we can be more aggressive in our approach. Forgetting DMSO, I take a conservative approach to any therapy that uses drugs in combinations. Too many safe drugs can become very toxic when mixed with other 'safe' drugs."

DMSO as a Controlling Mechanism with Autoimmune Disease

Central to the body's ability to defend itself against disease is its ability to produce chemical defending agents—known generally as antibodies. But when the body produces an excess of antibodies, the body's own defense forces can sometimes become internal enemies, interfering with basic life processes and attacking normal cells and tissues.

A number of serious diseases, including arthritis, cancer and even aging involve significant changes in the human autoimmune system. The disease known as myasthenia gravis, whose chief symptom is severe muscle weakness, is the result, it now seems, of an antibody attack against neurotransmitter receptors—minute structures in the nerve endings that link the nervous system to muscles. The attack prevents the neurotransmitter known as acetylcholine from activating the signal—from the nerve ending to the muscle cell—that underlies muscle movement. Studies now going on at Johns Hopkins University show that in rats, at least, DMSO has the ability to neutralize the action of the antibodies that produce symptoms similar to those in myasthenia gravis. However, it is much too early to tell if the same effect can be achieved in humans suffering from the disease.

It is clear from many studies that DMSO alters certain immunological responses, but the nature and implications of the effects are not yet well understood. It isn't known whether DMSO increases the activity of lymphocytes, the cells in the body that manufacture and secrete antibodies. It appears that DMSO's ability to relieve the symptoms of myasthenia gravis in rats is rooted in its ability to prevent certain antibodies from attaching themselves to neuromuscular junction sites. But it is also conceivable that DMSO is simply removing these antibodies from the body so that they never accumulate in sufficient concentration to bind themselves to the receptor sites in the first place. Robert Herschler refers to this property of DMSO as its "garbage collector" role: getting rid of self-manufactured agents that are causing problems.

DMSO as a Muscle Relaxant

The uniqueness of muscle tissue is that under normal circumstances, it can do one of two things, relax or contract. But sometimes, for any number of reasons, a muscle becomes physiologically unable to relax. This condition is commonly known as a spasm, or cramp. A study by W. Birkmayer presented at the Vienna Symposium on DMSO in 1966 showed that within an hour of topical application of DMSO, muscles in spasm show evidence of relaxation, as measured by an electromyograph. Clinical reports suggest that DMSO can quickly reduce the effect of so-called "night cramps"—the painful contractions that inexplicably strike people at night when they're trying to sleep. Some surgeons see promise in DMSO's ability to combat the involuntary spasms that often complicate surgical procedures, not because there are no effective tranquilizers that can produce the same effect, but because tranquilizers that act on the central nervous system can affect such functions as blood pressure, introducing still more complications.

DMSO's muscle relaxant mechanism doesn't appear to be directly tied to central nervous system functions. The most plausible explanation is that DMSO, by changing tissue permeability, rids muscles of undesirable metabolites associated with muscle work or contraction; here again, DMSO would be playing the role of a "garbage collector."

DMSO as a Cell Protectant

At the same time that Robert Herschler and, subsequently, Stanley Jacob were discovering the beneficial medical properties of DMSO, English scientists were discovering that it had value protecting a number of different mammalian tissues and diverse cell types from the damaging effects of freezing, freeze-storing and rapid thawing from very low temperatures. DMSO is routinely used throughout the world in laboratories involved in cryobiological research. It also shares with several substances, among them cysteamine, the ability to protect cells from the effects of X-rays and other kinds of radiation. A number of cancer centers in different parts of the world are beginning to use DMSO during radiation therapy as a way of protecting healthy cells that are ordinarily destroyed in the normal course of such therapy. DMSO has *both* radioprotective (against radiation) and cryoprotective (against cold) properties.

DMSO: Some Practical Considerations

Physicians familiar with DMSO stress time and again the fact that it isn't like other medical compounds. "There's a certain art to administering DMSO," points out Stanley Jacob. "You have to figure out the best way to use the substance individually with each patient you work with. Some people will respond to 70 percent DMSO solution but may develop a slight rash, so you have to weaken the concentration a little. In more serious conditions, you might elect to strengthen the solution. Sometimes topical application isn't the answer. One has to use injections— or maybe mix DMSO with another drug."

The average person who manages somehow to secure DMSO, either through a veterinarian or on the street, has little idea of how to use the substance, which is why Jacob, as well as other physicians who use DMSO in their practice, urge everybody who wants to use DMSO to always use it under a doctor's supervision. "I'm convinced it's a very safe drug," says Jacob, "but you have to know how to work with it. It takes a certain amount of experience and expertise the average person doesn't have."

All of which produces an interesting "Catch-22." For most doctors not only don't know much about DMSO but are reluctant to treat patients with it until such time that the FDA approves it for broader use. So even if you acquire DMSO and want a doctor who can supervise its application, you may not be able to take the substance under a doctor's supervision—not unless you're willing to travel to Oregon or some other place where doctors are more knowledgeable about DMSO and more willing to work with it.

With this dilemma in mind, and repeating again that you should do your best to find a doctor willing to supervise your taking of DMSO, here are a few general pointers to remember:

1. *Make certain the DMSO is pure.* This is not easy to do, since nearly all the DMSO sold on the black market today is commercial grade DMSO and could conceivably carry impurities that might cause adverse reactions. The fact that so few adverse reactions have been reported over the past year, despite the number of people using commercial grade DMSO, suggests that the danger of "impure" DMSO making you seriously sick is slight. Still, you're much better off with the DMSO approved for veterinary use or the 50 percent DMSO, which is the legally approved DMSO, for humans.

2. *Go easy at first.* To date, there has been no confirmed record of anyone suffering serious injury or death after taking DMSO. Occasionally a patient may be allergic to DMSO. To find out, rub a small amount of DMSO on the skin. If it produces any-

thing more than a redness or slight itching, it could mean that you're allergic and shouldn't be using it.

3. *Don't use DMSO stronger than 70 percent.* It looks as if the most effective DMSO solution strength for most types of pain relief is the 70 percent DMSO, which is 70 percent DMSO and 30 percent water. Higher concentrations of DMSO are likely to produce more redness and itching at the application site, but without necessarily producing an increased amount of pain relief. Fair-skinned and redheaded persons may have to reduce the solution strength somewhat. In any event, if any rash or other allergic reaction shows up on any part of the body other than the site of application, you should discontinue using DMSO.

4. *Stick with topical treatment.* Even though some people do report relief of many conditions by drinking DMSO, you shouldn't take it orally—unless a doctor has so prescribed it. If you're not one of the small minority of people who are allergic, you can safely use one-half ounce or so of DMSO two or three times daily on the skin in the area of your ailment, depending on the severity of the condition. DMSO tends to work better when you use *more* of it than when you use less, and it also works better when you apply it to an area considerably wider than the point of pain.

5. *Avoid contact with pesticides or other toxic materials.* Most veteran DMSO users apply DMSO to an area, let it penetrate for about fifteen minutes, and then dab the area even dryer with a towel. Usually the DMSO will be absorbed beyond the surface of the skin in about twenty minutes after you apply it. Although DMSO does have the power to carry with it into the skin materials that wouldn't normally go through the skin, the only danger you have to concern yourself with is direct contact with

a known toxic material, such as an insect spray or gasoline. Once the DMSO has dried and is no longer on the surface of the skin, its carrier properties are vastly diminished.

6. *Try not to use it every day.* Clinical experience shows that DMSO works best when you go off it for a day or so every now and then. One of the schedules that some chronic pain sufferers follow is to use DMSO for five days and then to go off it on the weekend.

7. *Expect taste and odor effects.* Most—but not all —people get a funny taste in their mouth when they take DMSO, and many people develop a breath odor that isn't always very pleasant. These two effects, apart from a temporary redness or itching on the skin, are the only two widely reported side effects connected with DMSO, and in years to come will probably be reduced by newer DMSO formulations already in use in Oregon. There is little that the average person can do to reduce these effects since the DMSO is simply enhancing the odors and taste that already exist in your body; but experienced DMSO users say that the taste and odor are diet-related.

"You have to recognize," Stanley Jacob urges, "that DMSO is not an easy substance to use. That's why I'm against the whole idea of people buying it illegally and using it on themselves. The drug needs to be approved for more uses, more doctors have to learn how to use it. We have to conduct a lot more research in order to tap the ultimate potential of the drug. If I had my wish," he adds, "it would be for at least $250 million for research to show how DMSO, in all its various forms, can help people suffering from conditions for which there is currently no safe and effective treatment. The potential for the good DMSO can do is enormous."

CHAPTER III

DMSO: The Athlete's Best Friend

Early one morning in June, 1963, a young Crown Zellerbach Chemical Products Division research assistant named Neil Frederick was heading down the stairs that led from the foyer of the company's research building to his basement office. When he reached the last step, his foot caught the edge of the stair. He fell, turning his ankle. "I knew I'd hurt it badly as soon as I fell," Frederick remembers. "But I limped into the office anyway. By noon, the ankle was very swollen and giving me a lot of pain."

Frederick's supervisor at the time was Robert Herschler, and Frederick knew of Herschler's preoccupation with DMSO. Frederick, too, had been intrigued by the chemical and by what Herschler was discovering about it. So he wasn't surprised when Herschler suggested that he put

DMSO on his sore ankle. Removing his shoe and sock, and using his hand as an applicator, Frederick rubbed a little DMSO over the entire inflamed area until it was dripping wet. Within fifteen minutes, he would recall years later, the pain was gone. "I could move the ankle without any pain. I didn't do anything else to the ankle for the rest of the day, and I walked around without pain or discomfort. I put the DMSO on the ankle again the next morning, even though the pain and swelling had disappeared, and neither the pain nor the swelling ever returned again."

Neil Frederick was one of the first of a long and still growing line of people who have experienced firsthand one of DMSO's most dramatic properties: its ability to cut the pain and swelling of sprains and other soft-tissue injuries as fast as if not faster than anything else available for such use.

Some eighteen years after Frederick's fall, a forty-two-year-old Connecticut man tried to change directions too quickly on a tennis court and fell, his left ankle stretching sharply and painfully under his weight. "I've had ankle sprains before," he says. "And this one seemed bad enough to keep me off the tennis court for at least a month." The difference with this sprain, however, was that the man saturated his ankle for three days with a 70 percent DMSO solution. "I used it the way a lot of athletes use it," he says. "I applied it not just to the ankle but to the whole foot, and clear up to the mid point of the leg. I did it every three or four hours. When I got home from playing tennis, about a half hour after spraining the ankle, I could hardly step on the foot. Two hours after I put the DMSO on, it didn't hurt anymore," he says. "I had some tenderness over the next couple of days, but I could walk without limping. If I had wanted to risk it, I could have probably played tennis three days later. I waited for five days. The ankle and leg felt a little weak, but I had no pain. I'll never know how severe the sprain might have been, but I have a feeling that if it hadn't been for the DMSO, I might have been out of commission for a good month."

Neil Frederick isn't sure how DMSO relieved his sprained ankle so quickly, and the Connecticut man is equally mystified. But their reactions weren't much different from the reactions of Robert Herschler when he first began experimenting with the drug on himself, on his pets, on friends, and on members of his family.

"I wasn't sure of what was happening," Herschler now says. "But I knew one thing: DMSO could do a lot of things no other substance I knew about could do."

Herschler feels more strongly about this today than ever. "The FDA keeps telling us that no one yet has *proved* the effectiveness of DMSO," he says, "but I'm willing to bet everything I own that, given enough time, I could get thousands of sworn statements from people who have personally experienced dramatic benefit from this chemical. If that doesn't prove effectiveness, I don't know what does."

Were Herschler to actually go out and begin soliciting such statements, his best bet would be to go to anyplace where athletes gather. For athletes—professional and amateur alike—have been swearing by DMSO ever since the early 1960's.

"My thumb was swollen to the point where I could not bend it," Daryle Lamonica, the former Oakland Raiders quarterback, testified at a Senate subcommittee hearing in July, 1980. "I took DMSO, there was a slight blister, but the swelling went down before my eyes. I couldn't believe it. Within five or six minutes, my skin was back to normal, and the majority of the swelling was down." Asked by the senators how DMSO differed from other treatments he might have taken for the same injury, Lamonica didn't hesitate. "Time" he said. "The difference was time. A pro-

fessional athlete isn't blessed with time where you can go
take two or three weeks from an injury."

Another witness that morning was Sam Bell, head track
and field coach since 1969 at Indiana University. Bell, at
one time the coach at Oregon State, has been recommending DMSO to his athletes since the early 1960's, but only
after he'd experimented with DMSO on himself, treating
an old ankle injury that swelled up badly whenever it was
slightly sprained. "Within three days," he says, "the swelling was down. I had no swelling, no soreness, no discoloration."

Bell's most memorable experience with DMSO involved
a young jumper named Daryl Horn, who had a shot at
making the U.S. Olympic team in 1964 but suffered a massive hamstring pull on the Monday before the weekend
trials. Horn was so black and blue and so sore that he
didn't even bother to travel from Palo Alto, where he was
training at the time, to Los Angeles, where the trials were
being held. Bell persuaded him to fly down anyway, met
him at the plane (Horn was limping so badly he could
hardly get down the portable stairs that led from the
plane entrance to the ground), and literally bathed the
jumper in DMSO for two solid days. "He didn't make
the team," Bell says, "but he competed and he only missed
qualifying by a half inch. He didn't come back to where
he was before the injury, but the fact that he was able to
compete at all was a miracle."

It's impossible to estimate just how many such "miracle"
stories have taken place in sports since athletes began using DMSO in the early 1960's, mainly because the majority of athletes who use DMSO choose not to talk about it
in public. "Sure I use it," one highly ranked professional
tennis player says, "a lot of guys on the tour use it. For
things like bursitis and tennis elbow, it beats aspirin and is
a hell of a lot better than getting a needle jammed into

you. But there's so much publicity about drugs and sports already that most players keep quiet about it."

But not all athletes are as reluctant to talk about DMSO. "I use it," says Dan Issel, of the National Basketball Association's Denver Nuggets. "It works a lot like deep heat, except it's much faster and heals much better than deep heat does." Former Portland State University quarterback Neil Lomax freely admits he's used DMSO throughout his football career, and Atlanta Falcons quarterback June Jones goes so far as to say that if it weren't for DMSO, he probably wouldn't be playing professional football.

"What I like about DMSO," says Al Oerter, the forty-five-year-old discus thrower who is the only American ever to win four gold medals over a sixteen-year period in Olympic competition, "is that you don't have to interrupt your training everytime you get a minor pull or sprain." Oerter, who gets his DMSO from a veterinarian and reduces it to 50 percent, says he uses it as an all-purpose liniment and has never had any adverse side effects. "I've never seen what all the controversy is about," Oerter says. "It doesn't pump you up like certain pills. It's simply a very useful thing to use for simple athletic injuries. Some people have told me that you shouldn't use it because it might mask the pain of a serious injury, but a good athlete knows his body well. Even when I'm using DMSO, I know when I can push and when I can't."

Not only athletes are high on DMSO, trainers and sports physicians like it as well. Graham Reedy, for instance, was first introduced to DMSO when he became the team physician for the Oakland Raiders and found that many of the players had gotten DMSO from jockeys at the Golden Gate Race Track, near Berkeley. "We used a 70 percent solution," Reedy says. "We would apply it liberally over an injured joint or muscle, let it dry for five minutes, apply it again, let it dry, and do this procedure four times a day for three to four days." Reedy adds that anytime a player was injured seriously enough to be hospitalized, he included the DMSO treatment with other modalities. The player's injured arm or leg was immobilized, iced and elevated for forty-eight-hour periods.

In Reedy's view, DMSO works best when you administer it for three to four days after an acute injury to a muscle or joint. The most dramatic effect he himself observed with DMSO occurred after one Oakland player, Bobby Moore, suffered a severe elbow contusion in a typical pile-up. "We put the DMSO on the elbow immediately after the game," says Reedy. "The swelling went down so quickly we could actually *see* it coming down." Reedy's experience, based on estimates from various players, was that players who took DMSO for acute injuries experienced a 50 to 75 percent quicker return to play than was seen with previous similar injuries not treated with DMSO.

Reedy says he tried for a time to test the effectiveness of DMSO in a controlled, double-blind-study manner. In a double blind study, neither the patient nor the doctor knows what drug is being used, only the *effects* of the drug. He made up two preparations: a 70 percent and a 10 percent DMSO solution. The experiment didn't work. The first time he treated Fred Biletnikoff with two different concentrations—the 70 percent DMSO on a sore ankle, and the 10 percent DMSO on a sore shoulder—Biletnikoff knew instantly which was which. "Doc," Biletnikoff snorted, "the stuff on my shoulder isn't the real stuff. My shoulder isn't red, and the stuff is drying too fast."

Not that Reedy found DMSO, in *any* concentration, 100 percent effective. Some 20 to 30 percent of the players he used it on had only minimal effect from its use, and for no explainable reason. "Maybe," he says, "it is an idiosyncrasy to accept or reject the drug." He also found that the drug wasn't noticeably helpful in chronic pain or joint disabilities, adding however, "we may not have given it a good try. We abandoned the use of the drug very soon when we experienced minimal response and had read that it wasn't as effective in chronic injuries." Reedy's conclusion: "DMSO, at 70 percent concentration, is an excellent drug that seems to significantly shorten the rehabilitation time for sports injuries to soft-tissue or joint defusions. It would definitely make a significant contribution to the fields of sports medicine, private practice and industrial medicine."

Most likely DMSO's ability to bring such quick and dramatic relief from acute muscular injuries is the result of its multiple properties. DMSO not only relieves the pain and inflammation that occur in sprains, it cuts down the swelling, relaxes the muscles around the injury and, as recent animal studies suggest, may actually help to shorten the healing time for injured cells. "Conventional treatments for sprains and similar injuries work in very limited ways," points out Stanley Jacob. "Ice can reduce the pain and swelling for a while, but it doesn't speed up the healing process, and ice doesn't increase the flow of blood to the injured area," he explains. "Pain-killers can relieve the pain but don't do much for the swelling and inflammation and don't help the healing process either. What's good about DMSO is that it reduces pain, cuts down the swelling, relaxes the muscles, increases the blood flow—and, at the same time, seems to promote the healing of injured cells."

Jacob also contends that DMSO is safer to use in athletic injuries than pain-killing agents like novocaine, which produce a numbness. "An athlete who receives a novocaine injection into an injury before competing," he says, "runs a much greater risk of aggravating the injury than an athlete who uses DMSO. The DMSO reduces pain, but doesn't make an area so numb that you lose touch with it. That's a crucial difference."

Whatever the principle of its action, the thing that athletes like most about DMSO is the speed with which it brings relief and promises healing. "When you're earning your living in athletics," Daryle Lamonica says, "you don't have the luxury of time. A non-athlete who gets a sprain can afford to nurse it for a couple of weeks and let time take care of the healing process. In athletics, a couple of weeks can mean the difference between having your job, or having somebody else in your position."

The speed of the therapeutic effects of DMSO has led Dr. Marvin Paul, a member of the University of Toronto Faculty of Medicine and former team physician to the Toronto Maple Leafs, to describe it as "the most important therapeutic agent available for the types of injuries so frequently encountered by athletes in competitive sports." Dr. Paul did a good deal of research in the mid-1960's, comparing results he obtained with DMSO treatment on various soft-tissue injuries with similar injuries he'd treated with conventional forms of therapy in 1964 and 1966. As a parameter of the efficiency of DMSO and the other therapies, he used the disability time produced by the injury. "The results," he says, "were startling. The disability time of an injured athlete who'd been treated with DMSO was a small fraction compared to the conventional treatment."

Dr. Paul even used DMSO on himself, for a recurrent slipped disc, and says without equivocation that "DMSO works better than anything else I have ever tried before or since DMSO therapy." He considers DMSO a superior treatment to other agents normally used in muscle injuries (not to mention the disc problem he himself has had throughout his life), because it allows the user to remain reasonably active throughout the healing period. "Time is going to clear up most soft-tissue injuries in spite of what you do," he says, "so all that physicians can do is give symptomatic relief, waiting for nature to take its course. I myself don't like to use pain-killers unless someone is against the wall," he explains. "The conventional way to treat a patient with a disc problem is to give an anti-in-flammatory agent and a muscle relaxant, but the problem is that if the muscle relaxant is going to work, you have to give such high doses that the patient gets drowsy and wants to stay in bed, which psychologically is a bad place —they get too used to it. DMSO combines both the effects of anti-inflammatory drugs with a muscle relaxant, and gives better results than when you use either anti-in-flammatories or muscle relaxants alone," Dr. Paul points out, and adds that besides this, "you don't get the serious side effects."

Considering all these glowing endorsements from athletes about DMSO's ability to heal certain types of injuries faster than anything now available, it's logical to wonder why the average person who suffers this kind of injury and wants DMSO has to get hold of the drug illegally. It's not a simple question to answer, but basically it comes down to the fact that, according to the FDA, nobody has yet done a carefully controlled study that *proves* the effectiveness and safety of DMSO. But Herschler and Jacob maintain that the FDA, because of the position it has taken on DMSO since 1965, has, in effect, *prevented* the very kinds of tests they are demanding. "Besides," Jacob says, "there were careful studies conducted in the early 1960's that the FDA to this day has never acknowledged."

One of the studies that Jacob cites was conducted by J. Harold Brown, a physician from the state of Washington, who reported his findings at the first New York Academy of Sciences DMSO Symposium, in 1966.

Working in a clinical setting, Dr. Brown randomly divided seventy-five patients suffering from a wide variety of strains, sprains and acute attacks of tendinitis and bursitis, as they came in for treatment, into three groups. He treated one group with an 80 percent DMSO gel. Another group he treated with a 10 percent DMSO solution (a solution that gives off the characteristic DMSO taste but doesn't have the anti-pain and anti-inflammatory power of the stronger solutions). He gave the third group a variety of what he called "standard therapy"—heat, oral analgesics, muscle relaxants and injections of corticosteroid medications.

Dr. Brown found, in general, that DMSO was noticeably more effective than any of the other therapies he used in his study—so much so that in his report on the study he stressed the difficulty he faced returning to what he referred to as "antedated treatment, namely oral analgesics, muscular relaxants, tranquilizers, corticosteroids, and physical therapy." He noted that the gratitude of the patients he treated with DMSO was "substantial, particularly since results were so promptly noticed."

What J. Harold Brown found in his studies in 1966, several other researchers conducting FDA-approved studies are now confirming, albeit nearly two decades later. Bob Reese, the trainer for the New York Jets, got personally involved with one such study after observing the effect that DMSO had on a deep thigh bruise suffered by linebacker Greg Buttle. From the appearance of the injury, Reese says, "it looked as if Greg would be lost to the team for two or three weeks. We started applying DMSO on Wednesday and by Sunday, Buttle was ready to play. I became a DMSO believer."

Reese's enthusiasm for DMSO resulted in the New York Jets becoming one of several professional sports teams participating in a study being done in conjunction with Young America Corporation of Connecticut, which has made DMSO available to the Jets—in both a liquid and a gel form—in exchange for test results. During the 1981 season, Reese estimates that he treated roughly two-dozen players, and he came to the same conclusion about DMSO as Graham Reedy: DMSO works extremely well with soft-tissue injuries—such as sprains, strains and bruises—and somewhat less effectively for chronic injury problems. "We had all the players diagnosed by a doctor before we used the DMSO," Reese says. "And we had written permission from all players before using it. We were careful about using it in cases where the chance of re-injury might be great—such as with torn ligaments. But for the things it worked on, it worked very dramatically."

On the strength of these and other studies, a 70 percent DMSO gel solution, to be used in the treatment of soft-tissue injuries, may get FDA approval by the summer of 1982. It will be prescriptive, and will carry detailed instructions on how it is best to be used. The fact that it has taken so long to get FDA approval of DMSO for these conditions is regrettable, but, as Herschler and Jacob point out, is symptomatic of virtually everything that has happened to DMSO since the early 1960's.

Still, not all physicians and athletic trainers, it should be said, are entirely pleased with the prospect of 70 percent DMSO becoming more readily available. Not because DMSO doesn't work effectively, but rather because it might work *too* well. Their worry is that a person who suffers an athletic-type injury and has some DMSO in his medicine chest might not take basic precautions, like having the injury checked by a physician or having it X-rayed. Another concern is that somebody treating himself with DMSO might decide to resume normal activity before the injury has healed sufficiently, and therefore stands a good chance of reinjuring himself—this time more severely.

"The fact that an injury no longer hurts or isn't swollen doesn't mean that the injury is *healed*," warns one New York physician. "When you sprain an ankle, for example, it takes a while, even after the symptoms are gone, for the muscle tissue in the lower part of the leg to regain its former strength. A person who tries to test that injury could very well aggravate the injury," he explains.

Stanley Jacob doesn't disagree. "Anytime you have any sort of acute injury," he says, "you have to take basic precautions. You check with a doctor. You get an X-ray. There's no question, either, that time is the safest healer of most soft-tissue injuries. DMSO doesn't replace time. It just helps it along."

CHAPTER IV

===============

When the Pain
Keeps Getting Worse

For three years prior to the Sunday evening his brother watched the *60 Minutes* segment on DMSO, sixty-year-old Sol Feinstein, a textile merchant from Minneapolis, lived in virtually constant pain. Two operations for a disc problem had left a legacy of scar tissue at the base of his spine. He had become, as he describes it, a "semi-invalid." As long as he rested frequently, didn't stand for too long a time and didn't try to do anything even remotely strenuous, he could manage, but any of the things he enjoyed —playing golf, taking long walks, riding a bike—were out of the question. "I'd start to walk for a while," he recalls, "and I could feel the pain start to build. I would get it in my legs, and it was like a bad toothache. It would get so bad I wanted to cry. If I kept walking, in spite of the pain, my knee would eventually buckle. I was a walking basket case."

Feinstein tried virtually everything to ease the pain. Aspirin was useless. High-power pain-killers worked for a time, but took away all his energy. "They made me feel goofy," he says. "Acupuncture helped."

Feinstein was one of the first persons to travel to Portland after the airing of the *60 Minutes* broadcast. He didn't know what to expect, he says, but he was desperate to find some way of living a normal life again. "I was impressed with Dr. Jacob," he says. "He was very low-keyed. He didn't *promise* anything. He told me he had a different approach. He told me if I gave it time, it might help."

Feinstein received several injections of DMSO, and when he got back to Minneapolis, he began a treatment procedure that Stanley Jacob no longer recommends because, as Jacob says, it uses too much DMSO. Each morning, at about 5:30 A.M. Feinstein would fill a bathtub with six inches of hot water. Then he'd pour 70 percent DMSO into one of those little totes that you put over your shoes in bad weather. He'd slip into the totes and soak his feet for at least half an hour. Afterward, he'd dump out the DMSO that was left and go about his daily business. He did it every morning.

"Dr. Jacob told me not to expect any real relief for at least a few weeks," Feinstein says, "and he was right. But I didn't give up hope. I figured if there was a chance the DMSO could help me, I was going to give it the full chance."

Within three weeks, in a gradual way, Feinstein began to notice a difference. The pain was still there but it wasn't as sharp, and it didn't come as quickly as it usually did when he walked. He could drive for longer periods of time. He found himself spending less time resting. He *felt* a little stronger, more positive about life in general. "With me," he says, "the relief wasn't overnight, but it was steady. Once I started feeling better, it was as if everything was turning around. I would walk somewhere and expect the pain to come, but it didn't come. I would be doing something at work, lifting sample cases, and I would surprise myself that I could do it without any pain. I kept asking myself if it was my imagination—if maybe the whole thing was in my head. I didn't realize, until I started getting better, how much I'd come to accept pain as a permanent part of my life."

Within ten months of his first DMSO treatment, Sol Feinstein was playing golf again, walking three or four miles at a time without pain, even riding a bicycle—something he thought he'd never do. He no longer had a slight stoop in his walk. "My doctor couldn't believe it," he says. "As a result of my condition, my right leg had atrophied so that it was an inch shorter than my left. Now, with all the walking and exercise I could do, it was back to normal again. Maybe it sounds corny to say it, but I think I owe my life, literally, to Dr. Jacob and DMSO. To live the way I was living before, with all the pain and with all the fatigue—it's not really living. The only way I can describe the feeling I now have is to say that I've been reborn."

If Sol Feinstein were the only person to maintain that DMSO has given him a new lease on life, one could dismiss his testimony as one of those medical "flukes"—something you can't really explain in medical terms, something that doesn't prove anything about DMSO one way or the other. But there are hundreds of people like Feinstein, people who lived with chronic pain for years, who suffered with the pain, who exhausted every conventional therapy, who'd been told by doctor after doctor that there was nothing, short of narcotics, that would ease their pain —and who have experienced dramatic relief from DMSO.

Consider Leona Whitney of Tualatin, Oregon. In 1973, she suffered a ruptured disc and spent four months in a hospital bed with what she describes as "the most agonizing pain possible." A year later, following months of tests and therapy, she underwent a second operation to repair a second ruptured disc. This time, the surgeon clipped some of the sensory nerves in an effort to stem some of the pain, but the pain didn't go away. "I couldn't live a normal life," she says. "I loved my work. My husband and I owned a garden and flower shop, but I couldn't go there anymore because of the constant pain."

More consultations with doctors led to a decision for yet another operation. "They wanted to take out three lower ribs," she says. "And I was ready to let them do anything. And that was when DMSO and Dr. Jacob came into the picture." She canceled the surgery and went on a DMSO therapy program, under Jacob's supervision. "I noticed relief by the second week," she says. "By the end of the second month, I was back doing all the things I used to do. The only time I have any pain anymore is when I do heavy lifting."

Then there's John Patrick Potter, a husky Portland blue-collar worker who, prior to coming to the DMSO Clinic, had been told by several doctors that nothing could be done for the scar tissue that had accumulated around his sciatic nerve as the result of two laminectomies—back operations in which vertebrae are fused. Like Sol Feinstein, Potter found that any time he walked for a while, his knee would suddenly buckle and he'd fall to the ground. He began walking with a cane to protect himself. "Before I started taking DMSO," he says, "I was on muscle relaxers, and a considerable amount of Tylenol, mixed with codeine. None of it was helping very much. The orthopedists I was going to told me that they could operate again, but also told me that in another year to year and a half, the scar tissue would form again and I would be back in the same situation. It wasn't a very encouraging prognosis."

Potter learned about DMSO through a friend who'd been coming to Jacob for treatment. For the first four weeks of Potter's treatment, he received only topical applications of DMSO, and didn't experience much relief.

Jacob then changed his strategy, and began administering injections under the skin. "After the third injection," Potter says, "I leaned my cane up in the corner. After the sixth injection, I quit taking the Tylenol and codeine. After twenty-four injections, I was completely pain-free."

The chronic pain that haunted Sol Feinstein, Leona Whitney and John Potter, and affects who knows how many tens of thousands of Americans, is a condition with no true medical classification. Pain itself is not a disease, but a symptom of many diseases; it is also a phenomenon that no one in science today fully understands. We know that pain is necessary—that without it, we would be denied one of nature's most basic protective mechanisms. Pain, after all, is what tells you to let go of a hot pot handle before it scalds your skin. It's the signal that tells you that a turned ankle hasn't healed enough to walk on.

On the other hand, for a great many people, pain serves no function other than to make them prisoners of their own bodies. Exact figures are hard to come by, but some estimates put the number of people in the United States who suffer from one form or another of chronic pain in the tens of millions. Some have chronic back pain. Others get savage migraine headaches. Others get terrible pain in the tips of their fingers whenever they do something as routine as reaching a hand into a refrigerator. Amputees experience pain—known as "phantom limb pain"—in a missing limb. Paraplegics and quadriplegics experience pain in areas of the body they can't move.

"Pain is one of the most mystifying conditions in medicine," says Stanley Jacob. And, he adds, "the biggest problem with treating it is that it's next to impossible to separate the pure physiology of pain from the psychology of pain. People have different physiological thresholds to pain. People also have different psychological thresholds to pain," he explains. "You never know, when you're treating a patient, how much of the pain is in the body, and how much of it is in the mind. Usually, it's in both places."

Hundreds of experiments bear out what Jacob says. Studies throughout the 1950's, for instance, suggested that, among other things, when you anticipate the onset of pain, you tend to experience it more intensely than you would if you were not anxious about its possibility. This explains why going to the dentist is such a punishing experience to so many people even in this age of novocaine and water-cooled drills. "Pain," observes physiological psychologist Ronald Melzack, "is a perceptual experience whose quality and intensity are influenced by many things: the unique past history of the individual, by the meaning he gives to the pain-producing situation and by his 'state of mind' at the moment. It's a very complex phenomenon to study scientifically."

Take a mystifying phenomenon like pain and mix it with a mystifying compound like DMSO and you get a subject that by no stretch of the imagination lends itself to succinct explanation. But several things can be said about pain and DMSO with a fair degree of certainty.

To begin with, DMSO *is* a highly effective analgesic, as clearly shown in a recent study done by two pharmacologists at Emory University in Atlanta, H. J. Haigler and D. D. Spring. Working with laboratory rats and using two measuring techniques for testing the analgesic effects of potent pain-killing drugs (in one of these tests, a rat is put on a hotplate and the time it takes before it starts to lick its paws is measured), Haigler and Spring found DMSO as effective a pain reducer as morphine. They found that the analgesic effect of DMSO lasts from two to four hours *longer* than that of morphine, and also found DMSO's analgesic effects unhindered by the anti-narcotic substance naloxone, indicating that DMSO doesn't operate on the addictive principle of narcotics. This last finding has been borne out time and again in clinical situations, for the longer you use DMSO, as opposed to most strong pain re-

lievers, the *less* of it you need to use to achieve a significant pain-reduction effect.

The precise nature of DMSO's pain-reducing capability
is still not clear. DMSO does have the power to inhibit
the transmission of nerve impulses by so called C-fibers,
neurons that are characterized by their relatively slow
impulse-conducting pattern and their high threshold—the
magnitude of the stimulus that is needed to set off an
impulse in them. Some physiological psychologists at one
time theorized that pain was simply a more intense inner
response to pressure, linked directly to C-fiber activity.
But there are too many aspects of the pain experience that
can't be explained by this simple cause-and-effect theory.

A new theory, known as the Melzack and Wall "gate-
control theory of pain," connects C-fiber activity with the
actions of other cells that connect to the brain and serve to
inhibit the firing of the C-fibers. And if, in animals, you
destroy the spinal-cord fibers that connect to these other
pain-related cells, the cells lose much of their inhibitory
power. This results in a sudden increase in the sensitivity
level of the C-fibers. This phenomenon might conceivably
explain a number of nonspecific pain syndromes in humans, especially those seen in the victims of spinal-cord
injuries, since the destruction of certain spinal-cord fibers
may prevent the firing of cells that function to inhibit the
firing of C-fibers. Under such circumstances, the C-fibers
might become supersensitive, permitting almost any sensation to set them off. Some researchers theorize that acupuncture may work on this principle—by activating the
cells that inhibit the C-fibers, thus cutting down the pain
that C-fiber activity induces.

If the ability to inhibit the firing of C-fibers were the
reason for DMSO's capacity to reduce pain, what would
explain the puzzling fact that DMSO is less effective in
chronic than in acute pain conditions? Neither Jacob nor
Herschler knows, and neither does anybody else who has

worked with DMSO. "It's a surprising phenomenon," says Jacob. "We'll get a patient who strains his shoulder and within an hour after we give him DMSO the pain is gone. We'll get another patient with chronic pain in his shoulder, and it may take five or six weeks before DMSO produces any lasting relief. Our rule of thumb here at the clinic, with any chronic pain condition, is 'don't expect any lasting relief for at least six to eight weeks.'"

Despite Jacob's downplaying of DMSO's power to ease chronic pain symptoms, dozens of DMSO clinic patients report almost overnight relief with DMSO from a pain condition they had lived with for years. Ann Clow is a twenty-seven-year-old former Portland woman who endured more than five years of almost constant pain after accidentally putting her fist through a window and damaging several of the nerves in her hand. High-powered pain-killers didn't help, and neither did two operations. "The only thing that helped," she says, "was soaking my hand daily in DMSO." Scott Tricarico, a 25-year-old New Bedford, Massachusetts, man suffered constant back pain for eight months following a car accident in 1975, and was in so much misery at times that he had to use support braces. DMSO brought him relief in a matter of days. Many of Dr. Jacob's patients report that they suffered so much pain before they began taking DMSO that they often contemplated suicide, and one patient, who says, "I now believe in miracles," went so far as to play a game of Russian roulette with himself.

But one of the most dramatic DMSO success stories to date involves an eighty-five-year-old New Yorker named Murry Becker. Becker—one of the oldest patients ever treated at the Portland DMSO Clinic—suffered for thirty years with short but severe bursts of pain that would virtually strangle the calves of his legs. In 1972, his condition was diagnosed as an atrophying spine, and he was told by doctors at Columbia Presbyterian Hospital in New York that there was nothing he could do for the condition, and that there was no really "safe" way in which he could control the pain. His physician prescribed Percodan, a powerful pain-killer. "Even the Percodan helped only intermittently," Becker says. "It took a half hour to take effect," he explains, "and it would hold me for about two hours. Then the pain would start all over again. There was just nothing to do about it, except struggle through it."

A successful New York lawyer who sits on a number of boards of directors throughout the country, Becker first came to see Stanley Jacob in June, 1980, more than three months after watching the *60 Minutes* program. "The most dramatic thing in the world happened," recalls Becker. "I walked in; I had all of my medical records, and after studying them, Dr. Jacob told me that at my age I couldn't expect the cells in my spine to come back. But he also told me that he'd had some success with pain that originates in the spinal area. He gave me some DMSO and told me how to use it.

"I went back to the hotel and used it that night," recalls Becker. "I used it the next morning, and that morning, I had an appointment with Dr. Jacob at eleven o'clock. Before I went to him, I walked from the Benson Hotel to the Meier and Frank Department Store, which I would say is about six blocks, and I did some shopping and walked back to the hotel. This was more walking than I had done in years."

As of this writing, Becker has never taken another Percodan or even a Bufferin, and insists that he has little or no pain. "I use DMSO twice a day," he says. "I rub it everywhere from my waist down. I've been to my personal physician and he's given me a full battery of blood tests —the results were all negative. I'd heard about certain eye problems, so I promptly made an appointment, when I got back from Portland, with my eye doctor. He told me that my eyes were no worse than they ever were, and if anything might have been a little better."

Stanley Jacob can offer no definitive explanation for Murry Becker's "overnight recovery," other than to suggest that it might have something to do with DMSO's effect on collagen. "We know," he says, "that DMSO can soften scar tissue in the body, but it usually takes a long period of time. Maybe in some cases, all it takes is a little softening for pressure on the nerve to ease."

An equally dramatic story, in its own way, involves a concert organist from Portland named Lorraine Miller, who insists that if it weren't for DMSO she would either be an invalid or dead. A polio victim at the age of eighteen months, Lorraine lived the first eighteen years of her life in a back brace, but nonetheless became an accomplished organist. A few years after the brace was removed, she began to experience horrible pain throughout much of her body—a problem that was eased a good deal by an operation that fused some of the vertebrae in the middle of her back. Several years later, however, the pain again returned—this time even more punishingly. "It would hurt so bad when I would wake up at night," she says, "I felt like throwing up."

Like so many victims of chronic pain, Lorraine went from specialist to specialist and was ultimately advised that the only way her pain would go away was if she underwent yet another vertebrae fusion, this time at the top of her spine. Such an operation, however, would have made her a virtual invalid. She would have needed the constant care of her adopted daughter, whom she alone— as a single parent—was raising. And she would have been forced to give up the organ entirely. These prospects were so grim that Lorraine Miller seriously talked about suicide to her priest. "I saw no point to living," she says, "one way or the other."

At last report, after being on DMSO therapy for several months, Lorraine Miller was experiencing less pain than she could remember experiencing since her body brace came off more than twenty years earlier. She was giving concerts (some of them to benefit DMSO research) and teaching. "If somebody had told me when things were the blackest," she says, "that someday I would be putting in twelve- and thirteen-hour days without suffering pain and without getting exhausted, I wouldn't have believed them. I'm not ashamed to say that I owe DMSO my life."

Equally puzzling to Jacob is the success he has had in treating patients with ureteral stones. The ureter is the tube that carries urine from the kidney to the bladder. Occasionally, it gets clogged with gelatinous, insoluble substances and calcium, forming stones. "It's a very painful condition," explains Jacob, "and you can't explain the pain relief by simple C-fiber activity." Jacob's guess is that by inhibiting cholinesterase, DMSO produces a peristalsis effect. That is, it produces rhythmic movements in the muscles within the walls of the ureter, forcing the contents to move. This enables some patients to pass the stones on their own.

What is especially curious about DMSO's pain-relieving capability is its ability to reduce pain in conditions for which other pain-killing agents are not usually effective. The pain that affects people suffering from certain forms of terminal cancer, for instance, is unresponsive to all but the most powerful narcotic drugs—such as morphine or heroin. Yet DMSO can be remarkably effective in relieving such pain—so much so that former Indiana governor Otis Bowen, a physician, rubbed DMSO on his wife, who at the time was dying of multiple myeloma, a deadly type of bone cancer. Bowen made national headlines when he admitted to a gathering at an American Medical

Association conference that despite the FDA position on DMSO, he had obtained the substance from a veterinarian, had used it on his wife and had been able to relieve his wife's pain, he said, "in minutes." "The bottle said 'for horses only,'" Bowen says, "and we laughed together, but it really wasn't funny." He then asked the audience: "Why can't dying persons with severe pain have easy prescription access" to DMSO?

The frequent ability of DMSO to alleviate the constant pain that compounds the tragedy of paraplegia and quadriplegia explains why former Alabama Governor George Wallace was a patient at the DMSO Clinic, in Portland, for two weeks during the summer of 1980. DMSO can alleviate the burning and constant pain suffered by people who have had the disease known as shingles. It has long been considered by many physicians that if the pain associated with shingles persists for longer than two years, it becomes a pretty much permanent and incurable part of a person's life, even if the shingles themselves don't return. But Stanley Jacob has treated at least two patients whose pain from shingles had been going on for more than two years, and found that the newer formulations of DMSO brought relief to both.

Still, not *all* types of pain respond equally well to DMSO treatment. Migraine headaches, for instance, don't generally respond well to DMSO, most likely because of DMSO's vasodilating effects—its expansion of blood vessels whose pressure against structures in the brain may account for migraine pain in the first place. Jacob has found, too, that topical applications of DMSO are only occasionally successful in relieving pain in the hip joint or in the knees, although he has had better success treating these patients with DMSO injections.

"When it comes to certain types of pain," Jacob says, "we'll probably get the best results with DMSO mixed with other drugs, but as a general all-purpose pain reliever, all things considered, DMSO is the best thing around, in my view."

One of the many people who wouldn't disagree with this assessment is Naida Carlson, of Seattle, Washington, for whom aspirin, cortisone shots and other anti-inflammatory agents did little to ease the severe pain of a bursitis condition in her shoulder. "The medical folks kept telling me that because I was fifty years old, I was just going to have to learn to live with these kinds of infirmities for the rest of my life," she says. "But somehow I just can't believe that God would intend to keep us alive just so that we can suffer. DMSO took the pain out of my shoulder the first time I used it."

CHAPTER V

═══════════════════

The Arthritis Question

When you are a seventy-two-year-old widow, living alone and on social security, the last thing in the world you need is rheumatoid arthritis in your hands. "After a while," says a Philadelphia woman named Rose, "you just give in to it. I've had shots, I've taken pills, I've lived on aspirin. Mostly they just made me groggy and sick. So what you do is try to adjust to it. I don't go out when it's cold. I don't try to do anything like sewing with my hands. Some days I'll just sit and soak my hands in water and watch the game shows. It's not much of a life—but you get used to it."

People like Rose are at the root of much of the controversy that has bedeviled DMSO over the past two decades. For a basic question about DMSO from the beginning, has been how much hope it holds out to persons suffering from arthritis—chronic joint and connective-tissue inflammation disease that plagues nearly 32 million Americans.

Although not as lethal as heart disease or cancer, arthritis is nonetheless the third most prevalent cause of disability in the United States, ranking in this respect behind only heart and circulatory diseases and mental illness. It can strike in any of 100 different forms, from relatively mild "aches and pains" to savagely degenerating forms that cripple, maim and eventually lead to death. And it exacts a particularly hard toll on older people—serious enough in 40 percent of cases to require a physician's attention. The impact of arthritis on the American economy —when you add up the medical expenditures, lost wages and lost manpower hours—comes to about $10 billion a year. And this doesn't take into consideration the cost of the illness in human suffering. By any measure, arthritis is a medical problem of monumental proportions.

Because arthritis is a chronic disease, patients who have it are usually on a steady regimen of medicines, and pharmacological research into the disease has sought to develop drugs that can relieve the pain and inflammation of the disorder but are mild enough in their side effects to allow safe, long-term use. It has been an elusive search. There are dozens of anti-inflammatory drugs on the market today, but it is the rare patient who can take any of them for any length of time without eventually developing a tolerance to the drug's anti-inflammatory effects, or experiencing a wide and often disruptive range of side effects—from skin rashes and blurred vision to temporary short-term memory loss. In some cases, the drugs may even prove fatal. And although many arthritic patients rely mainly on aspirin for pain relief, aspirin has its shortcomings as well.

"Setting up a drug treatment regimen a patient can live with is one of the biggest problems in treating arthritis," says Dr. Arthur Scherbel, chief of rheumatology at the Cleveland Clinic Foundation. "A lot of people—particularly older people—can't even tolerate aspirin. It causes gastric irritation if they take it in large doses. Elderly people with impaired hearing have added hearing problems when they take large doses of aspirin. The idea," he says, "is to try and find various ways of using a combination of drugs that we have in our therapeutic arsenal. Certain patients notice a greater effect from one drug. Other patients have more effect from another drug. There is nothing simple about this disease."

All of which brings us to DMSO. On the basis of its fundamental properties, DMSO would appear to be an ideal arthritis medication. It is an excellent pain reliever. It is anti-inflammatory. It is something you can use topically, applying it directly to the area that hurts. It is, furthermore, inexpensive, and its minor side effects make it suitable for long-term use. So, given these properties and given the scope of the arthritis problem, you would think that an arthritis patient asking the simple question, "Can DMSO help my arthritis problem?" should be able to get a simple "yes" or "no" answer. Not quite.

The arthritis patient who wants an objective answer to this question invariably meets a conflicting—and frustrating—pattern of responses. "I don't know *who* to believe," a Florida woman who has had a troublesome arthritic knee for nearly ten years said two months after she saw the *60 Minutes* DMSO segment. "I have friends who swear by DMSO, but my doctor doesn't know about it, hasn't tried it and doesn't believe in it. I watch a television show that seems to tell me that the drug might help me, but the information I get from the Arthritis Foundation tells me it might be dangerous. I'd like to try it, but I'm afraid of it."

Complicating the basic question of whether or not DMSO is an effective arthritis medication has been the sudden appearance over the past year or two of arthritis "DMSO clinics," chiefly in Mexico but also in Florida, Nevada, and elsewhere. The treatment at these clinics consists, in the main, of a series of shots, generally given over a thirty-day period, but also available by the week.

The treatment is expensive—as much as $2,500 for a month's worth of injections—and it is reported that in some of the Mexican clinics, the injections aren't *pure* DMSO, but DMSO mixed with anti-inflammatory drugs. The problem with these treatments isn't so much their effectiveness (many patients do indeed report obtaining pain relief), it is that some clinics lack professional medical supervision, and lack of supervision poses a threat to a patient who could react adversely to the drug being mixed with the DMSO.

It's no secret, of course, that tens of thousands of arthritis patients are now treating themselves with commercial-grade DMSO, purchased in various ways on the DMSO black market. "I cut it down to about 65 to 70 percent strength," explains an Ohio truck driver who uses DMSO for an arthritic condition in his lower back and buys it from a local source as a "solvent." "I rub it on all over my lower back and buttocks when I first get up in the morning," he says, "and I can usually drive all day without much discomfort. I know somebody who pours the DMSO in a pan, soaks his hand in it for about ten minutes and then pours the DMSO that's left back in the bottle."

Not surprisingly, many rheumatologists—physicians who specialize in arthritic diseases—are dismayed that so many arthritis patients are treating themselves topically with DMSO or else seeking treatment at DMSO "clinics." The Arthritis Foundation, in its publications, has done its best to scare people away from DMSO, creating the impression that DMSO is no different, really, from any number of "quack" cures and nostrums that have come down the arthritis pike over the years and have done little but engorge the bank accounts of the promoters behind them. "Much of the enthusiasm for DMSO," claims Frederick McDuffie, senior vice-president for medical affairs of the Arthritis Foundation, "comes from testimonial, not from scientific data. This is a pattern physicians and researchers

have come to expect whenever new 'miracle' pain reliev-
ers are announced, and it is why even quack remedies can
enjoy brief periods of public attention." McDuffie goes on
to warn arthritic patients who are taking DMSO that they
may be endangering themselves by ignoring "proven
forms of treatment." "Arthritis can't be cured," he acknowledges, "but modern treatment methods—medication, physical therapy, surgery—are highly effective in
controlling pain, in preventing damage to the joints and in
enabling arthritis patients to live happy, productive lives."

Maybe so. Perhaps many of the arthritis patients currently treating themselves with DMSO are not consulting
their local rheumatologist as frequently as they should, not
taking as many drugs or receiving as many shots. And
there is no question that the victims of severe and chronic
arthritis conditions, most of whom are older and on fixed
incomes, are vulnerable to unscrupulous promoters who
offer limited prospects of relief at a high financial pre-
mium. But even if Dr. McDuffie and his colleagues at the
Arthritis Foundation are sincere about the welfare of arthritis patients, he still paints a distorted picture of the
relative role that DMSO is *now* playing in arthritis treatment and should continue to play as the years move on.

First of all, according to a poll taken by staff members
of Representative Claude Pepper, from Florida, who
heads the House of Representatives Select Committee on
Aging, Dr. McDuffie's position on DMSO is by no means a
universal view among American rheumatologists. Prior to
the March, 1980, hearings on DMSO and arthritis, the
Pepper Committee sent out a questionnaire to a random
sampling of 250 rheumatologists. Of the 68 percent who
responded, 20 percent said they had used or prescribed
DMSO in their practice, and about 50 percent of this
latter group felt the drug was "effective in reducing inflammation, pain or other arthritic symptoms." Interestingly, too, about 15 percent of the physicians who had no

experience with DMSO expressed the feeling that it was indeed "effective" in reducing inflammation.

More troubling, however, is the impression created by Dr. McDuffie that—DMSO apart—the so-called "proven forms" of treatment are a legitimate avenue of relief for everybody who suffers from arthritis. Dr. McDuffie fails to mention in his attack on DMSO what every rheumatologist surely knows: that for a substantial proportion of arthritis patients, especially those with rheumatoid arthritis, the "proven forms of treatment" not only fail to bring effective relief but produce uncomfortable and often debilitating side effects.

Consider three of the most widely used non-steroidal, anti-inflammatory drugs—Naprosyn, Motrin and Clinoril. Each of these drugs is generally considered effective but each carries troublesome side effects. For instance, according to the *Physicians Desk Reference* (PDR), Motrin will produce adverse gastrointestinal reactions in 4 to 16 percent of patients. Roughly one in seven persons who take Naprosyn, according to the PDR, can expect adverse gastrointestinal reactions. With Clinoril, the proportion of patients who report adverse reactions is somewhere between 8 and 15 percent. Among the side effects reported with all of the drugs are headaches, fatigue, stomach upset, blurred vision, asthma and a number of central-nervous-system reactions ranging from "psychotic episodes" to coma.

But side effects apart, the current array of arthritis medications hardly represent *ideal* therapy. A 100-pill bottle of Clinoril (200-milligram strength) costs anywhere from thirty-five to forty dollars. And most patients develop a tolerance to these drugs: the longer they take them, the more it takes of the substance to produce relief (and the greater the likelihood of side effects).

Yet another "proven treatment" some rheumatologists would have their patients seek out rather than a substance as "unproven" as DMSO is gold salts. Introduced in the 1920's, gold salts received the status of a "proven treatment" largely on the basis of a double-blind study conducted in 1971 that showed that 77 percent of rheumatoid arthritis patients given these salts experienced subjective and objective improvement, with 23 percent reporting an apparently lasting remission.

That's the good news. The bad news (apart from the fact that nobody has any idea of how gold salts work) is that one out of five persons who receive gold injections responds with a serious allergic reaction—so serious that many rheumatologists won't administer gold salts at all. Gold is a highly toxic substance, potentially lethal if a doctor miscalculates the dosage schedule; and even under closely monitored conditions, it interferes with the body's ability to manufacture leukocytes—the white cells whose primary function in the body is to resist infection. "The gold injections devastated me," says one woman from Pittsburgh who now reports excellent results with DMSO that she applies topically to her hands. "I broke out in a horrible rash from the gold injections. I couldn't walk for days. My blood platelet levels fell so much, I had to take iron and B-12 injections for several weeks. All told, I was out of commission for a good two months, and it was three or four months before I felt myself again. At the end, my arthritis was no better—it was worse."

Nobody is more aware than Stanley Jacob that every "proven treatment" in arthritis—even aspirin—produces its share of uncomfortable and potentially dangerous side effects among a certain proportion of the people who take them. This is not because Jacob is a rheumatologist, but because virtually all of his Portland, Oregon, DMSO Clinic arthritis patients are battle-scarred veterans of conventional therapies. "People come to *us*," Jacob points out, "not because they're neglecting conventional therapy, but because they've had conventional therapy and it hasn't helped. We get the true 'end of the line' arthritic patients, and we're producing significant relief in about 70 percent of the cases."

Typical of the "end of the line" arthritic patient who has sought out the DMSO Clinic at the University of Oregon Health Sciences Medical Center is Harris York, a stocky and amiable former shipyard worker in his early sixties, who has suffered from a steadily deteriorating arthritic condition in his back, arms and legs over the past twenty years. The source of York's problem was diagnosed in 1979 by a Tacoma doctor as a "deteriorating spine." X-rays showed an accumulation of sediment, from the deterioration at the base of the spine, that had "locked" on a nerve. The pain, York described, was excruciating and constant. "I couldn't do anything," he says. "I couldn't sit, stand, lie down or find a place for myself. I couldn't sleep for more than thirty minutes, and then I'd be up because of the pain. And nothing they gave me helped, either. None of the drugs. None of the therapy. Nothing."

York's Tacoma doctor offered him one of two options. The first was to take narcotics to kill the pain. The other was to undergo what his doctor described as a "good-sized" operation, whose results he could not guarantee. "Well," says York, "I didn't have the money for an operation, and I didn't want to start on narcotics. I'm not smart to begin with so I don't want to start messing with drugs that might affect the way that my brain works."

A week after his depressing consultation with his doctor, York read in his local paper about a young paraplegic in the state of Washington who was being helped by DMSO therapy. "I figured," he says, "that if something is good enough to make a paraplegic start to move, the stuff has got to help me."

York put in a call to the DMSO Clinic, pleaded for an appointment, and made his first visit to the clinic in November, 1979. "Dr. Jacob didn't promise me anything,"

York says. "He told me that if the DMSO was going to work, it was going to take time. I told him not to worry, that I'd been hurting for twenty years and that another couple of months wasn't going to kill me."

Jacob began treating York with injections of DMSO, just under the skin, three times a week. York says he got the DMSO taste in his mouth and the odor, but felt no relief until one morning a month after his first injection, when he woke up for the first time in ten years without pain. That relief, however, was short-lived. "Very short-lived," says York.

The injections continued, as did the topical applications that York would administer to himself twice a day. By January, 1980, York was beginning to feel better. "You have to understand," he says, "that everything is relative. When you're hurting for so long, you're grateful when you're only half hurting." By February, 1980, York was responding so well to the treatment that he needed fewer injections. Instead of visiting the clinic three times a week, he was coming now once every few weeks, while continuing to use DMSO topically. "I went from having almost constant pain," Harris York says, "to almost *no* pain. My life is livable again. We could use more money in my house, but you can't reconcile money with pain, so I'm not complaining. My life is worth living again. As far as I'm concerned, DMSO is the most wonderful drug I have ever heard tell of."

Harris York is not a scientist, or even a college graduate, but he has a quick and pragmatic mind. You're not going to get very far with him by suggesting he is incapable of evaluating the effectiveness of DMSO. "There is nobody in the world," he says, "going to convince me that I'm imagining things. I've had every pill you could take for arthritis, and the only thing that ever worked for me has been DMSO."

Most of the arthritic patients who have come to the

DMSO Clinic over the past several years share Harris York's opinion. A former editor of *The New Yorker* magazine who has lived in retirement in the Portland area for the past fifteen years insists that he is by nature a highly skeptical person, but that DMSO is the only drug he's ever taken that has effectively relieved the pain of his gout condition. "The only thing I know," he says, "is that thanks to DMSO I'm playing golf again."

A thirty-nine-year-old woman who earns her living decorating cakes says that if it weren't for DMSO, she couldn't work. "When I would get a rheumatoid arthritis attack," she says, "my fingers became so stiff and so painful I couldn't move them. Now I rub the DMSO on the joints of my fingers and hands, and I have virtually no pain."

A seventy-three-year-old St. Petersburg, Florida, man says that before he took DMSO, the arthritis in his shoulder was so bad he couldn't lift his arms. "Now," he says, "I can lift a bicycle over my head and put it on the garage rack. I never thought I'd be able to do this again."

But do such testimonials constitute legitimate scientific documentation for the effectiveness of a drug?

To many rheumatologists, such claims represent "religion," not "science." But there are several scientific studies that give credence to these claims. In the early 1960's, the Japanese Rheumatism Association carried out a study on 274 victims of rheumatoid arthritis, the systemic arthritis condition in which the inflammation takes a progressively crippling course throughout the body. The investigators divided the patients into three groups: one received a 90 percent DMSO solution; the second received a 50 percent DMSO solution; and a third received a placebo substance —propylene glycol. All of the treatments were topical. The results of the study showed that the patients receiving the 50 and 90 percent DMSO experienced what the investigators termed "significantly" more relief in joint pain and in range of movement than the patients in the placebo group. This study didn't show DMSO to be any more effective than *other* arthritis medications, but it determined that arthritis patients could get relief from DMSO and use it safely.

Other clinical studies show results similar to those of the Japanese study. German physicians Heinz John and Gerhard Laudahn reported, in their paper given at the 1965 New York Academy of Sciences Symposium on DMSO, that 80 percent of the osteoarthritis patients they treated topically with DMSO for a period of from two to six months experienced either a partial or complete remission of symptoms. They also reported that roughly 75 percent of rheumatoid arthritis patients experienced "significant" relief. Their study suggests that arthritic conditions in the spine and in the small joints respond better to DMSO treatment than do conditions in the hip and the knee. They also found that many patients received effective relief by combining DMSO with reduced dosages of their normal medication.

Clinical studies done for Syntex Laboratories in the early 1960's by Dr. Arthur Steinberg showed that chronic arthritis patients given topical DMSO applications four times daily experienced pain relief in about 84 percent of cases, and also demonstrated increased mobility and decreased swelling in the inflamed joint. Steinberg found that when DMSO therapy was discontinued, the swelling returned. His study also showed that rheumatoid arthritis patients experienced subjective pain relief from DMSO about 77 percent of the time, and, like Drs. John and Laudahn, he reported that several patients got relief from a combination of DMSO with a reduced dosage of their normal medication.

"We're not saying that DMSO can get to the underlying cause of any arthritis condition," says Stanley Jacob. "Its effects are definitely symptomatic. The chief benefit is pain relief and more mobility. Patients feel better. They can get around better. They manage the problem better with DMSO than with other drugs."

Jacob stresses the importance of proper administration of DMSO. He doesn't contend that DMSO works for every arthritis patient, but suggests that clinicians who have not reported success with the drug may not be using it properly. He also maintains that DMSO's ultimate role in arthritis treatment will be as an adjunct to other drugs. "With some patients," he says, "the topical DMSO works fairly well—as long as it's a strong enough strength—70 percent being what seems to be the ideal. But other patients do better on shots under the skin in the beginning, with the topical administration as a back-up," explains Jacob. "In any event, what we've found here at the clinic is that you achieve the best results from DMSO when you use a lot of it and apply it not just to the inflamed area but to a wide lot of the surrounding area as well." And he adds that "we've found that DMSO works better for arthritis above the waist than below the waist, and found that the most resistant part of the body to DMSO treatment is the hip."

Many rheumatologists will grant to Jacob that DMSO works to some degree as an analgesic (although some insist that DMSO is no more beneficial to pain relief than Ben-Gay or other over-the-counter analgesic ointments), but the degree to which DMSO reduces inflammation and, on a different level, inhibits the progression of the disease is another question.

Yet, here, too, there is a small but growing body of scientific evidence to suggest that DMSO does indeed reduce the inflammation that is at the source of many arthritic problems, and there is some evidence suggesting that DMSO is biochemically capable of stabilizing the condition. "We can't say that DMSO can *reverse* the progression of an arthritic condition," Jacob says. "But if you can keep a patient where that patient is—that's more than any drug can do right now. And I don't think I'm overstating the case when I say that DMSO might be able to do this."

Backing up Jacob's view that DMSO reduces arthritic inflammation is a study by two Hungarian scientists, Peter Gorog and Iren B. Kovacs, who gave to rats a form of arthritis whose inflammatory effects come closest to the inflammation that occurs in human rheumatoid arthritis. This was a very carefully controlled study in which the affected rats were divided into five different groups. One group received a 90 percent DMSO solution, the second, DMSO plus hydrocortisone, a third hydrocortisone ointment alone, a fourth no treatment, and a fifth group acted as a non-arthritic control group.

It is well known that hydrocortisone has a potent anti-inflammatory action, but most people have a very limited tolerance to this drug. The Hungarian study showed that while the hydrocortisone alone was more potent than DMSO as an anti-inflammatory agent, the local anti-arthritic effect of the hydrocortisone was increased tenfold when DMSO was used as "carrier." And the DMSO by itself, without any hydrocortisone, showed significant anti-inflammatory effects.

The Hungarian rat studies take on special significance when you compare the results with the reported results of a study done recently in Russia by a scientist named A. P. Aliabeva and two colleagues. Russian rheumatologists have been conducting clinical studies with DMSO and other substances since the early 1970's; this particular study, which ran from 1972 to 1978, was done to "determine the effectiveness of DMSO when used in combination with other medications for rheumatoid disease."

The Russian researchers treated 343 patients, 320 of whom had rheumatoid arthritis and 23 of whom had deforming arthritis. The majority of the patients were female, all between the ages of sixteen and fifty-two. Most had been suffering from rheumatoid arthritis for between three and five years and were in what rheumatologists call the second degree of the disease. Prior to the study, all the patients had been taking anti-inflammatory agents similar to those widely used in the United States.

The largest group in the study—145—received pure DMSO in a 50 to 70 percent solution strength. The DMSO was administered topically, directly to the source of inflammation. The rest of the patients received DMSO in combination with other substances. Eighty-five of these remaining patients—those suffering from the most pain—received DMSO and what is described in the study as an "analgin" (i.e., a pain-killer). Another fifty—those with significant inflammatory joint changes—received the DMSO with heparin—a substance produced by the body that is sometimes used to prevent blood clotting. Another twenty-five received DMSO mixed with sodium salicylate. Some of the patients were also given shots of cortisone throughout the study, although the shots were generally limited to the "more resistant" cases. The parameters used as criteria in the study were pain intensity, joint movement and the level of inflammation in the affected joints.

The results of the study show that 64 percent of the patients who received DMSO alone exhibited improvement, 19 percent showed "insignificant improvement," 15 percent showed "no effect" and 2 percent were described as worsening. With the DMSO combined with analgesic, the "improvement" percentages are slightly higher. The data regarding the patients who received DMSO along with hydrocortisone were judged to be insufficient to make any definitive conclusions. Only 3.2 percent of the 343 patients had side effects worth mentioning, and in most cases these side effects were confined to skin irritations at the DMSO application site.

"We may conclude," the Russian report says, "that the use of DMSO for inflammatory and degenerative joint diseases is well founded. The use of DMSO with other medications (heparin, sodium salicylate, hydrocortisone) increases their effectiveness, which in turn produces a quicker decrease in pain, exudate manifestations and other signs of joint inflammation; it also improves joint function. The fact that the dosages of anti-inflammatory medications can be decreased with the local use of DMSO is very important," continues the report. "Treatment with DMSO in different combinations is tolerated well by patients and side effects are seldom encountered."

But even more significant than the results of the Russian study are the findings of a study recently reported in the European Journal of Neurology (Eur. Neurol. 19:141 151 1980) by a group of Japanese physicians from the Department of Internal Medicine at Hiroshima University School of Medicine. The doctors were studying a kidney condition known as amyloid polyneuropathy, a kidney inflammation that sometimes arises in rheumatoid arthritis patients. DMSO not only produced clinically measured improvements in the state of the disease, but urine analysis of the patients revealed the presence of an increased excretion of low-molecular-weight proteins and a "remarkable increase of IgG and IgA excretions": antibodies produced—and in this case directed against the body itself —by the body's immune system.

The significance of this finding is that there is now more reason than ever to believe that the underlying cause of rheumatoid arthritis—indeed, the underlying cause of many collagen-type diseases—is an overproduction in the body of molecular autoimmunological agents known as immunoglobulins. Immunoglobulins are produced when the surface receptors on white blood cells (lymphocytes) interact with antigens. This interaction transforms the lymphocytes into so-called plasma cells, which then produce the five major types of immunoglobulins.

Since the blood serum of rheumatoid arthritis patients

shows high concentrations of certain immunoglobulins, it has been theorized that patients with this disease are hypersensitive to these as the rheumatoid factor—that is, their system produces disease-causing agents. Conceivably, the excess amount of these immunoglobulin combinations (as Rh factor) somehow leads to an excess of collagen build-up and other problems. Conceivably, too, DMSO, through its binding actions with the immunoglobulins, prevents this systemic build-up by increasing their excretory rate.

"It's much too early to make any definitive conclusions about DMSO's effects on anti-antibodies and the implications for rheumatoid arthritis," says Robert Herschler, "but the findings are very significant. They suggest that DMSO can play a kind of garbage-collector role in the body, getting rid of substances that would otherwise accumulate and cause trouble."

As for Stanley Jacob's overall conclusion about DMSO and arthritis, it is basically this: he doesn't see DMSO as a "cure" for any form of arthritis, but believes that for many arthritis patients it's a versatile, easy-to-use pain-relieving agent with a minimum of side effects. "People can manage their conditions better with DMSO," he says. He believes, too, that in serious arthritis cases, DMSO works best when used in combination with other drugs, although he says that much research is necessary to determine which combinations work best for different patients. "DMSO," he says, "is not the miracle arthritis drug that will ultimately solve the problem, but it's bringing substantial relief to most of the people who come to our clinic—and these are people who haven't been helped by other treatment. And not only do we find people getting relief, we find good reason to believe that their conditions *stabilize*. Therefore, says Jacob, "if it isn't the *ultimate* answer, it's certainly one of the options an arthritis patient should have."

CHAPTER VI

======================

To Save a Life

It happens on the average of once every ten minutes in the United States alone. An ambulance screeches to a halt at the emergency entrance of a hospital, often followed by a police car, its siren light making wide, lazy circles in the night. Within seconds paramedics or sometimes the police themselves are wheeling somebody into the anxious glare of the emergency room. In most cases, the injured person is a young man, frequently a teenager, who has been critically injured in a car or motorcycle accident. But sometimes it's someone who's been shot or hit over the head. His face is often blanketed with blood or horribly discolored, but sometimes you would swear he was merely sleeping. The nurses and physicians on duty know better, and you can sense the urgency.

Time, often the healer in medicine, is now the enemy. If the heart stops beating, the doctors and nurses still have two or three minutes to get it pumping again before the brain cells that control basic life functions run out of oxygen. If the brain or spinal cord has been damaged, every minute lost could mean the difference between somebody who lives and somebody who dies, between somebody who walks out of the hospital on his own two feet or strapped to a wheelchair he may have to live in for the rest of his life.

Stanley Jacob is as familiar with these gruesome, anxious scenes as anybody in medicine, because he's been there himself in the emergency room hundreds of times when victims of severe head and spinal-cord injuries have been rushed in for emergency treatment. So, when he talks about DMSO and its potential to save the lives and bodies of thousands of people each year who are either killed or paralyzed because of head and spinal-cord injuries, his voice takes on an added edge. "We used to think," he says, "that the damage caused at the moment of injury in a severe head or spinal-cord injury was irreversible. But now there are animal studies and a handful of clinical cases that tell us something different. There is still a little bit of time before the injured cells die. Based on what we've seen in animal studies and a handful of human situations, we think that if you can treat a head-injury victim within a few hours of the injury, or a spinal-cord victim within one hour, there is a good chance of preventing death or the paralysis that would otherwise occur."

That the range of DMSO's properties might save lives in hospital emergency rooms didn't initially occur to either Stanley Jacob or Robert Herschler when they first began working with DMSO in the early 1960's, but in retrospect the rationale seems clear enough. Severe injuries, particularly to the head and the spinal cord, almost invariably sabotage a number of basic life processes, among them respiration, blood pressure and blood flow; and here, the multiplicity of DMSO's properties gives it a range of therapeutic potential matched by no other drug currently being used in emergency treatment. But here again, we're faced with the dilemma of an effect without a clearly understood explanation.

"It isn't any *one* thing," says Dr. Jack de la Torre, who has pioneered in the research on the use of DMSO in head and spinal-cord injuries. "It's a combination of effects, any one of which could make a difference depending on the kind of injury. But the critical factor is *time*."

Dr. de la Torre began working with DMSO in 1971 as part of a search he and some colleagues, at the University of Chicago, were conducting for drugs that might be effectively used in treating head traumas, but within a year he expanded the scope of his work to cover spinal-cord injuries as well. De la Torre's experimental method is to induce in various species of laboratory animals—rats, dogs and monkeys—head and spinal-cord injuries that simulate in these animals the kind of devastating central-nervous-system damage that occurs in humans who suffer severe head and spinal-cord injuries. He then divides the injured animals into different groups, and gives each group a different treatment. Some of the animals receive drugs currently used in the treatment of these injuries, such as mannitol or heparin. Some of the animals receive nothing but a saline solution. At least one group of animals receives DMSO intravenously. De la Torre also varies the timing of the treatment, with some of the animals getting treatment within moments of the injury and other animals getting treatment after several hours. The important thing is that the injuries are the same in all the animals; only the medication and the timing of the treatment differ.

The first thing that de la Torre and his colleagues noticed when they began their work was that DMSO could reduce intracranial pressure quicker and more effectively than any of the other drugs they were using.

Intracranial pressure is the pressure that arises inside the skull when injured brain tissues swell, as the result of fluid leaking from damaged cells. A similar kind of swelling—or edema, as it is called—occurs when you sprain an ankle or a thumb. The difference, though, is that in areas outside the brain the skin can expand to accommodate the swelling. The skull doesn't expand, so that when edema occurs in the brain, pressure begins to build up. This increased pressure further damages the brain.

There is almost always some degree of intracranial pressure any time a person has suffered a head or spinal-cord injury, but its impact on the injury victim varies from person to person, according to the site and the extent of the injury.

Very often, the pressure will go down on its own, in time, and as long as it isn't too great or isn't affecting regions of the brain that control critical functions, a patient can withstand extended periods of abnormal intracranial pressure—for as long as forty-eight hours—without necessarily suffering any long-term effects. This is why you will frequently hear physicians attending a head or spinal-cord injury victim say that it may be a couple of days before they can tell for certain how much permanent damage the injury victim has sustained. They have to wait to see if the loss of a certain function is simply a temporary consequence of the pressure, or is the result of permanent damage.

On the other hand, if pressure builds in an area of the brain that controls critical functions—such as breathing or heartbeat—doctors don't have the luxury of time. They must reduce the pressure and do it quickly. Monitoring the pressure with a measuring device inserted directly into the skull, doctors have at their disposal a variety of means for reducing the pressure: they can use a drug called mannitol that is effective most of the time; they use steroids or barbiturates.

But there are times when none of these pressure-reducing measures work, and it is a foregone conclusion that if doctors *can't* control intracranial pressure, the patient's chances for survival or for a recovery free of permanent neurological damage are severely compromised.

"DMSO," says Dr. de la Torre, "was able to reduce intracranial pressure better than any other substance we were using. So, at this very early stage in our studies, we made what we felt was a very important discovery. Even if DMSO did nothing else but reduce intracranial pressure, it would be a very useful drug in the treatment of these kinds of injuries."

But de la Torre and his co-workers soon began to notice that DMSO was having other effects that boded well for victims of catastrophic injuries. They noticed, for instance, that the injured animals that had been given DMSO showed an increased flow of blood through the two blood vessels—the carotid arteries—that bring blood to the brain. This increased blood flow didn't occur in either the control animals or the animals on the other medications. And they found that within ten minutes of administering DMSO, the level of brain-wave activity in the injured animals, as measured by an electroencephalogram, become more active, a noticeable contrast to the flattening of the electroencephalogram that appeared in other animals just prior to death.

DMSO also demonstrated an ability to stabilize blood pressure in the injured animals—a crucial consideration in most head and spinal-cord injuries, since the inability to control blood pressure can lead to a patient's death. Injured animals treated with DMSO showed, as well, a deeper and faster breathing pattern than the other animals —still another beneficial effect, inasmuch as shallow and insufficient breathing are almost invariably complications in head and spinal-cord injuries.

Finally, de la Torre noticed that DMSO produced five times the urine output that other treatments did, indicating DMSO's ability to draw water from the injured tissues in brain areas that control basic life functions.

"What we were doing in these early studies, very simply," says de la Torre, "was comparing the effects of DMSO with other medications in certain basic functions that are always affected when you have a serious head injury."

These initial DMSO experiments led the University of Chicago group to expand their observations to central-nervous-system damage resulting from cerebral strokes and from injuries that produce permanent damage to the spinal cord. If you induce these injuries in animals, and you don't give any treatment, the animals become comatose or lethargic, or else die. In the case of a permanent spinal-cord injury, the animal becomes permanently paralyzed if you don't apply treatment.

De la Torre has used the same general procedures in these later studies that he used in the initial experiments. All the animals are given the same type of injury, but different forms of treatment. De la Torre and his colleagues then observe, measure and record the results.

"The first thing we notice when we give DMSO intravenously," says de la Torre, "is that there is an immediate increase of blood flow through the spinal cord to the region of the trauma." He points out that this increase is extremely significant, for one of the first things that happens in a severe spinal-cord injury is that the blood vessels constrict, reducing oxygen and blood flow to the injured area and preventing the flow, in and out of tissue cells, of enzymes and other materials needed by the cells to survive.

The clinicial manifestations of these experiments are striking and their results have been reproduced by researchers at the University of Pittsburgh, at Bowman Gray University and by other researchers at the University of Chicago. In experiment after experiment, in different types of injuries and in different species, de la Torre and his colleagues find that DMSO-treated animals fare consistently and dramatically better than animals that either receive no treatment or receive the medication routinely used in head and spinal-cord injuries in humans.

In one study involving thirty monkeys, all of which received identical head injuries, all ten that were given only a saline solution died, whereas seven of ten that received urea—a substance often used in the treatment of head injuries—survived, although three showed obvious neurological defects. Of ten monkeys given DMSO, however, every one survived, and only one showed any effects—a temporary paralysis of the right arm. De la Torre has seen similar results in various studies involving more than 500 monkeys.

In other studies, involving dogs, de la Torre and his co-workers have found that animals given DMSO shortly after receiving an injury normally known to produce permanent paralysis are not only spared paralysis but are able to regain almost normal function within a few weeks. The same recovery pattern does not materialize with dogs given a saline solution or with dogs given either mannitol or Decadron, two drugs that are standard treatment in central-nervous-system injuries.

Exactly why and how DMSO can minimize and in some cases virtually nullify the normally catastrophic consequences of these kinds of injuries is something nobody is quite sure of, but there are any number of plausible explanations. Certainly, the ability of DMSO to reduce intracranial pressure so quickly and effectively is one of the factors involved, but, as any neurosurgeon will tell you, there are many instances in which brain- and spinal-cord-injury victims die or are paralyzed regardless of how effectively you control the pressure. One possibility is that DMSO's ability to trap so-called free radicals—agents that trigger adverse reactions—may account for the stabilizing role it plays in central-nervous-system injuries.

Another interesting theory, backed up by preliminary animal studies, is that DMSO serves to protect the membrane of so-called glial cells. Glial cells are cells in the nervous system that do not themselves transmit signals but serve a supportive function: they hold the nerve fibers in the nervous system in place, and regulate the flow of energy-related material to the neural cells and of waste matter out of them. They also serve to insulate neurons (nerve cells) from one another, and remove dead or damaged cells from the nervous system.

DMSO's protective effect on glial cells could help to answer one of the most perplexing questions raised by de la Torre's research, as follows:

It has long been an established neurological principle that damage to nerve cells in the central nervous system, unlike damage to cells in other parts of the body, is irreversible. This would explain why a spinal-cord injury, for instance, can produce permanent paralysis, or why a stroke or head injury can produce permanent and often devastating consequences. One suspected reason for the inability of damaged nerve fibers to recover is that the axon of a neuron—the long extension that transmits impulses from the cell body to other neurons—is "starved" for the nutrients it needs by the scar tissue from damaged glial cells. If this is true—if the inability of an axon to regenerate itself is linked to the presence of scar tissue from damaged glial cells—and if it is true that DMSO can prevent additional damage to glial cells, we have at least a *theoretical* explanation for why DMSO might prevent the damage that otherwise occurs.

"What the animal data are showing us," says Stanley Jacob, "is that cells in the central nervous system that have been damaged in a head or spinal-cord injury might not be 'dead' at the moment of injury. If animals are given DMSO intravenously quickly enough, they survive and do not show some of the paralyzing aftereffects one would normally expect. It has been demonstrated repeatedly in monkeys by de la Torre that following injury, early treatment lessens destruction of cells. My suspicion is that not all the damaged cells 'die' immediately upon injury. You have a little bit of time to prevent their destruction."

Jacob is careful to point out that humans have a much more complex system than other animals, and that the difficulty normally encountered in establishing human applications from animal studies is therefore compounded when it comes to DMSO in these types of injuries. De la Torre, too, is careful when he talks about the relevance to humans of his animal studies.

"What we've shown in our studies," says de la Torre, "is that when animals have certain kinds of injuries that normally would either kill them or leave them paralyzed, DMSO can often prevent or reverse many of the pathological signs that occur. How DMSO works in these systems is still highly theoretical, but I think it has something to do with the capacity of DMSO to do a lot of different things—things that no other drug we know of can do. When you're up against any injury in which the central nervous system is involved," he explains, "you're faced with any number of different problems, any one of which can be fatal. As far as we've been able to tell, DMSO helps to stabilize many of the functions that can either kill or cause paralysis in animals."

For obvious reasons, research that might answer the question of whether DMSO can do for head- and spinal-cord-injured humans what it does in animals is scant. You can't very well gather a group of twenty people in a room, subject each of them to an injury designed either to kill or paralyze them and then administer a number of substances to see which substances prevent death and paralysis and which substances don't. What you have to do is wait until you've come across an injured patient in such terrible shape that no conventional treatment has produced any relief and *then* administer DMSO to check its effects.

Which, essentially, is what neurosurgeon Harold D. Paxton, of the University of Oregon Health Sciences Center, has been doing for the past year or two.

Paxton and his colleagues are studying the capacity of DMSO to do at least one thing in humans that Jack de la Torre has demonstrated in animals—reduce intracranial pressure very quickly. This capacity became apparent the first time Dr. Paxton and his colleagues tried DMSO. An emergency-room patient suffered a massive head injury, and the pressure had not responded to either mannitol, steroids or barbiturates for three days. Yet minutes after the patient received an intravenous injection of 40 percent DMSO, his intracranial pressure dropped down to a level that was no longer jeopardizing his life, and it stayed down. The patient died, but under the circumstances— the severity of the injury—Dr. Paxton and his colleagues felt that DMSO had proved itself and deserved more study. Three more patients with critical head injuries in whom mannitol, steroids and intravenous barbiturates failed to reduce intracranial pressure were given DMSO, and the original pattern repeated itself: the intracranial pressure came down, but the patients died anyway from the damage incurred at the time of the injury.

On the fifth try, however, the Oregon neurosurgeons not only succeeded in reducing the intracranial pressure of a patient suffering from a severe head injury, saving the patient's life, but, even more remarkable, enabled the patient to make a good enough recovery to be able to return to work as a respiratory therapist. "He survived in a situation where we otherwise would have predicted death—and not only survived, but recovered," says Dr. Paxton. "We administered DMSO six times over a forty-eight-hour period. Each time we were able to reduce the pressure to a level where it was no longer jeopardizing the patient."

Once convinced that DMSO could reduce intracranial pressure as well as if not better than other medications, Dr. Paxton and the other neurosurgeons he was working with decided it was time to use DMSO earlier in the treatment process in controlling intracranial pressure. In this phase of the study, patients who failed to respond to mannitol or steroids or hyperventilation were given DMSO instead of intravenous barbiturates. Six patients underwent the treatment and, here again, DMSO effectively reduced intracranial pressure in all of them. Three of the patients died despite the DMSO, and one of the survivors suffered with permanent neurological effects. But two of the patients not only survived but made what Paxton describes as a "good recovery."

Dr. Paxton is guarded in his conclusions. "At this point," he says, "we have shown what we set out to show—that DMSO can reduce intracranial pressure in some severe instances in which other drugs won't work. We're not sure *how* it does this, but I suspect it has something to do with its very strong diuretic properties." But although his team has had some patients who have survived, "we can't make any flat statement concerning DMSO in these types of injuries," he says. "Intracranial pressure is only one of the complications that arises in these injuries."

A clinical study similar to the study Dr. Paxton conducted in Portland is now going on in San Diego, at the University of California, under the direction of neurosurgeon Dr. Perry Camp. No one on the neurological staff is discussing publicly the protocol of the study until the

FDA has seen the results and made its decision. Even so, early reports out of San Diego suggest that Dr. Camp is highly pleased with the results so far. "We're monitoring results here, at the University of California at San Francisco, and at the University of Oregon," Dr. Camp was quoted by a San Diego *Union* reporter in January, 1981. "DMSO's use in the control of intracranial pressure has had encouraging results. We know from animal studies that DMSO has the potential to diminish some of the brain deficit that occurs in stroke victims. What we're trying to find out in this study, among other things, is whether DMSO might be used as a first agent for strokes. It might work, but it might turn out to be too dangerous."

Among the "dangers" that concern Dr. Paxton and other neurosurgeons working with DMSO in head-injury treatment is that intravenous DMSO in relatively large concentrations, 40 percent or higher, produces a condition known as hemolysis, the destruction of red blood cells.

What happens in hemolysis is that some blood cells leak hemoglobulin. This leakage discolors the urine. Increased bleeding time is a complication, although not necessarily a serious one. In any event, the neurosurgeons who are now working with DMSO have reduced the concentration to 10 percent, which lessens the hemolysis and bleeding-time problems. The effect of DMSO in such cases is "probably an osmotic effect," says Stanley Jacob. "We noticed it in the early studies and reduced the concentration. But one has to remember that we're dealing with catastrophic situations. The chances of a patient who's had a terrible head or spinal-cord injury dying because of prolonged bleeding time are much less than the chances of dying from the complications that DMSO may help to control. If I were being treated, I'd risk the blood problem, and ask for the 40 percent solution," he says; "it works faster."

Although it will be quite a while before all the results of the current DMSO studies on central-nervous-system trauma are in, there are a growing number of specialists in the field who share Jacob's belief. Sean Mullan, the chairman of the Dept. of Neurosurgery, University of Chicago, has given intravenous DMSO to nine patients with postoperative hemiplegia (partial paralysis). His conclusion: "DMSO is safe in the dosage used. It is probably effective in the very early stages of treatment of postoperative hemispheric effect. The present assessment is one of cautious optimism."

DMSO: How Much Hope for Paraplegics and Quadriplegics?

Given its ability to prevent paralysis from occurring in certain injuries where it might otherwise occur, it is a logical question to ask whether or not DMSO has the power to help paraplegics and quadriplegics *regain* neurological function that has seemingly been lost. Some paraplegics and quadriplegics experience spontaneous recovery within two years of their injury, but after two years it's almost universally accepted that somebody paralyzed because of a spinal-cord injury has gone about as far as he is going to go in terms of regaining any new function.

Stanley Jacob is unusually guarded when he talks about DMSO and its potential to help paralytics. Part of him wants to give paralytics and their families some ray of hope, but he isn't convinced yet himself just how much DMSO can do to help victims of spinal-cord injuries if they haven't been given the DMSO within an hour or so of the injury. "We've treated about fifty stabilized paralytic patients so far with DMSO," Jacob says. "None of them are walking, but there are some who honestly believe that they *will* walk some day, and as long as they have hope, I'm going to do whatever I can to help them. We've seen some improvement in quadriplegics that you wouldn't normally expect," he adds, "but it takes a long time and a lot of hard work on the part of the patient who's paralyzed. I

believe DMSO has a place in the rehabilitation of paraplegics and quadriplegics, but we're going to have to wait
and see just how far we can go with it."

Probably Jacob's biggest success story to date is a young
Edmonds, Washington, man named Mike Taylor, who was
all but killed in the mid 1970's in a motorcycle accident
that twisted his neck some 180 degrees, breaking it, and
leaving his head wedged against his chest. His parents
were told a day after their son was taken to the hospital
that the boy would never again have the use of his arms or
his legs. He would be a quadriplegic for life.

"The doctors advised my wife and me to put Mike in a
nursing home," recalls Mike's father, Lyle. "I had one doctor just about beg me to do it, insisting that if my wife and
I didn't listen, taking care of Mike would destroy all of us.
But there was no way that Barbara and I could do it. Mike
was our youngest child, and we were determined to de-
vote the rest of our lives, if necessary, to Mike's rehabilitation."

Lyle Taylor quit his job and went into the insurance
business close to home, so that he could have flexible
hours and spend as much time as possible at home, taking
personal charge, along with his wife, of his son's rehabilitation. "We'd set goals," he says. "If Mike could sit up in a
chair for two minutes at a time, that was a big deal. We'd
go for three minutes the next day. Mike was just fantastic.
He was a wrestler in high school and always had tremendous self-discipline, but I never realized just how tough
and great a kid he really was until we started on this program."

Taylor did everything a person could do to learn about
new techniques, new therapy, new drugs—anything that
might offer some hope to his son. He was even set to go to
the Soviet Union, which has a world-renowned paralysis
treatment center, but the doctors there refused because it

had been nearly two years since Mike's accident and they felt the Taylors would be wasting their time. The Russian trip fell through, so the Taylors took Mike to Stanley Jacob's DMSO Clinic.

In one of the nurse's offices in Jacob's DMSO Clinic, there is a Christmas card on the wall. It stays there all year. "Mike Taylor sent us this card," explains Rita Roake. "He signed it with his own hand."

Signing a Christmas card with his own hand (instead of with a prosthetic device) is only one of the things Mike Taylor can do since he began a program of intravenous DMSO, some three-and-a-half years after his injury. He's gained enough control of one of his arms to be able to operate his own wheelchair; but more remarkable, perhaps, is the change that has taken place in his "sensory evoked potential." The sensory evoked potential (SEP) is a test that measures the amount of electrical activity going on in an injured area of the spine. On August 8, 1977, Mike's SEP showed a normal response in the left median nerve, but no response at all in the right median nerve, which controls the left arm. Eighteen months later, there was activity in both areas and a suggestion of activity in the areas that control Mike's legs. The specialist who analyzed the reading wasn't quite sure what to make of it. And still isn't. Either "it's a natural variation in the somatosensory evoked response," he says, "or an improvement isn't clear at present."

Jacob, too, would have trouble accepting the fact that years after the injury that left him crippled, Mike Taylor is showing improvement in nerve function, were it not for another of his patients—Grey Keinsley, of Colorado, who also didn't begin DMSO therapy until more than two years after the accident that left him a quadriplegic. Keinsley, who was diagnosed a c-4 quadriplegic, is the only person on record with that diagnosis who has voluntary motor control over both of his feet. "He can't walk," Jacob says, "but even to be able to move his feet voluntarily, beginning several years after injury, is extraordinary."

Other paraplegics and quadriplegics on DMSO therapy have experienced less dramatic improvement but improvement all the same. Many paraplegic males, for instance, are able to have erections but suffer from a condition known as retrograde ejaculation, in which the sperm moves backward, into the bladder. DMSO, reports Jacob, has stabilized the condition in several of the patients he's treated. Paraplegics and quadriplegics on DMSO also experience fewer bladder infections, have fewer problems with bedsores and show a better ability to maintain their body temperature.

"The one thing we noticed about Mike after he'd been on DMSO for a while was that he seemed a lot stronger," says Lyle Taylor. "It used to be that a couple of hours in the wheelchair and he'd have to go lie down. Now he can stay up for fourteen or fifteen hours without any trouble. What it means is that he can live a reasonably normal life even with the handicap," explains his father. "He goes to school. He's got a business of his own. He can do a lot of things on his own that he never could do."

Whether Mike Taylor will ever leave his wheelchair under his own power—he is convinced he will, and spends four hours a day on physical therapy—nobody knows. Neither does anybody know for certain the role that DMSO is playing in his improvement. Some neurosurgeons, when told of Taylor's recovery, suggest that maybe there was some mistake in the beginning, when his injury was first diagnosed. What is curious about this is that some neurosurgeons and orthopedic surgeons refuse to even entertain the idea that DMSO might be doing something inside Mike Taylor's nervous system that nobody would have thought possible.

"*I* can't say what's happening," Stanley Jacob says. "It's possible that DMSO is simply stimulating cells that have been dormant but not dead. I certainly don't say that DMSO is bringing 'dead' cells back to life. But," he concludes, "neither can I ignore what I'm seeing with my own eyes."

It's true, of course, that Mike Taylor and Grey Keinsley are the exceptions among Jacob's quadriplegic and paraplegic patients; the majority have not done nearly as well as these two. But then who is to be the final judge of what "improvement" really means. "What most people have trouble realizing," says Grey Keinsley—who is now a successful insurance claims executive in Colorado—"is that what seems inconsequential to the average person may have monumental significance to somebody who is paralyzed. The fact that a person can comb his own hair or shave or partially dress himself. If DMSO can get a person just *that* far, it's done more than anything else can do, and it can make an enormous difference in a person's ability to get up each day and face the world."

CHAPTER VII

======

Mental Retardation and DMSO

Twenty-two-year-old Billy King, of Portland, Oregon, doesn't strike you as the sort of young man a mother would go out of her way to introduce to strangers. Mentally retarded since birth, he has the classic look of Down's syndrome: the slightly slanted, Oriental-like eyes, the flat nose, the small and stubby hands characteristic of mongolism. He can speak a few phrases, but you cannot carry on any sort of conversation with him. Yet, when you are invited into the home of Betty Lou King and her husband, whom everybody knows as "Speed," Billy is introduced to you early on. And if the Kings are self-conscious about having a retarded son, you would never guess it.

Not that the Kings are carrying out a charade. Betty Lou has no delusions about her son, who is her only child. She knows Billy will never be "normal" in the conventional sense of the word. She knows he'll never go to college, never pursue a socially prestigious career, never marry and never make her or her husband grandparents.

But won't waste your time feeling sorry for the Kings: you'd only end up trying Betty Lou King's patience. "When I look at Billy," she says, "it is not with pity. It's with love and with pride. And if you knew Billy ten years ago, you'd understand what I mean."

Billy King is one of an estimated 75,000 persons in the United States afflicted with the condition generally referred to as mongolism but more accurately described as Down's syndrome, after Dr. John Langdon Down, who first identified the condition in the 1860's. Billy is also one of a handful of Down's syndrome individuals on a drug therapy program involving DMSO. For the past ten years, Billy King has been receiving injections of DMSO, mixed with chemical substances that activate nerve function and are known as neurotransmitters—the protein units that play a fundamental role in the process by which neurons transmit information to one another. Some specialists attribute the developmental and behavioral problems of mentally retarded individuals to a lack of neurotransmitters in the central nervous system. When injected on their own, however, neurotransmitter chemicals do not seem to pentetrate many of the central-nervous-system areas for which they are targeted. When given in conjunction with DMSO, their penetrating properties are greatly enhanced.

"It's still hypothetical," explains Stanley Jacob, "but there is a great deal of animal data to back up the hypothesis. We know that certain neurotransmitters can stimulate brain function in animals. We know that when you combine these neurotransmitters with DMSO, you see better penetration into the brain and a greater density. What remains to be seen is how much this type of therapy can do to change the developmental patterns and the behavior of severely brain-damaged people."

As far as Betty Lou King is concerned, "hypothetical" is a meaningless word. When her son began DMSO therapy at the age of thirteen, he was underdeveloped even by Down's syndrome standards. He was also at an age—although Betty Lou didn't know this at the time—at which most children with Down's syndrome have long since passed the peak of their social and intellectual development. Billy, she says, was a "loving child" and a relatively well-behaved child, but he was virtually helpless. He couldn't dress or wash himself, couldn't control his bladder or his bowels and could barely understand the simplest of instructions. And not because he hadn't been given special attention. "We went everywhere and tried everything with Billy," Betty Lou says. "He had the best special schools, the top specialists. We even had a speech therapist on a regular basis for years. We tried different drugs; nothing helped. What Billy used to do most of the time was listen to the stereo and bang his head up against it in time to the music."

Today Billy King not only does many things on his own that he never used to be able to do, like control his bladder and bowels, dress himself and eat at the table in a mannerly way, he can also swim the length of an Olympic-sized pool, can understand most basic instructions and can verbalize things he could never verbalize before. No longer does he sit for hours banging his head against a stereo.

He works for half a day each day during the week at a special employment center for the mentally retarded, where the workers put airline music and movie headsets into plastic bags. "Do you want to know what parental pride is?" says Betty Lou King. "It isn't watching your son graduate from Harvard. It's receiving in the mail a social security card with the name of a teenager who, only a few years before, couldn't even go to the bathroom by himself. That's pride."

To say that Betty Lou King is grateful for what DMSO has done for her son is an understatement of monumental proportions, and much of her gratitude is directed toward Stanley Jacob and much also to a remarkable scientist-businessman from Chile named Nicholas Weinstein. Weinstein, who died recently at the age of eighty, was a Ph.D. chemist at twenty who founded and ran Chile's largest private pharmaceutical firm, Recalcine. Stanley Jacob, who met Weinstein in 1971, describes him as one of the most unusual and impressive men he's ever met. "It wasn't only that he was brilliant," Jacob says, "he had a very deep sense of humanitarianism."

Weinstein and Jacob met face to face for the first time in 1971, and Jacob recalls the excitement in Weinstein's voice when they talked about DMSO. "Weinstein told me that from the moment he read the first paper on DMSO, he was intrigued by the chemical. He felt it was the most important pharmaceutical development in his lifetime."

Chile has its own version of the FDA, but it grants medical researchers and drug companies greater latitude than the FDA to conduct clinical studies, particularly in conditions for which there are no known cures. Weinstein had a special interest in mental retardation as well as other central-nervous-system afflictions. His interest stemmed from the fact that CNS pharmacology, despite its remarkable development, holds little prospect for measurable therapeutic improvement in patients with such afflictions. Weinstein sensed immediately the implications of DMSO— that its mysterious ability to penetrate, with apparent safety, regions of the brain inaccessible to nearly all other non-toxic substances might have a revolutionary impact on the pharmacological therapy of such central-nervous-system disorders. He developed a number of new chemical formulas in which powerful substances of known effectiveness were combined with DMSO but at a much reduced level, the better to cut down on their toxic side effects. He donated huge amounts of these new substances to hospitals, nursing homes and institutions for the chronically ill. One of the new formulas he helped to develop combined DMSO with three neurotransmitter amino acids, aminobutyric acid (GABA), amino hydroxybutyric acid (GABOB) and acetylglutamine. And this combination, a substance known as Merinex, is the one Billy King has been taking since 1971—as well as being the substance used in a major clinical study that took place in Santiago and Valparaiso in the early 1970's, under the control of nearly a dozen of Chile's most prominent specialists in infantile neuropsychiatry, pediatrics and neurology.

The study involved fifty-five children, all of them fourteen years old or less. All were diagnosed as having trisomy-21, the technical name for Down's syndrome. The condition is called trisomy-21 because of the idiosyncratic chromosomal make-up of Down's syndrome children. In normal persons, all of the cells in the body contain forty-six chromosomes, arranged in twenty-three pairs, or "sets." But for reasons nobody knows, all of the cells in persons with Down's syndrome contain an extra, forty-seventh, chromosome. And it is this extra chromosome, which links up, as a third chromosome, to the two chromosomes in the twenty-first pair, that accounts for the name trisomy-21. Although this "extra" chromosome is normal, it interferes with the cell's ability to duplicate itself in a way that insures orderly growth and development.

Nobody involved with the Chilean study, least of all Nicholas Weinstein, had any delusions about "curing" the children. Trisomy-21 is genetically induced, and therefore always present in the cell that is the product of conception—and consequently in every other cell in the body of the human being that grows from that single cell. In a certain sense, to "cure" trisomy-21 would require reversing a pattern of incalculable complexity—in every cell of the body.

On the other hand, all of the investigators who took part in the study were reasonably convinced that if DMSO could, in fact, take certain amino acids into areas of the central nervous system where these substances could not penetrate on their own, they might be able to activate "suppressed" neural function, and in so doing bring about some measurable improvements in development and intellectual function.

The complexities in such a study are staggering. First of all, there is no uniform rate of development among Down's syndrome children, and there is good reason to believe that nutrition and environment go a long way to shape their behavorial and social development. Numerous studies suggest that Down's syndrome children raised at home (where, presumably, they are given more personal attention and love) develop more quickly than institutionalized Down's syndrome children. They walk at an earlier age and they tend to be more verbal when they grow up. Few specialists are willing to state unequivocally that Down's syndrome children raised at home will grow up to be "happier" than institutionalized children, but whatever their mental and physical limitations may be, children afflicted with the syndrome are no less psychologically sensitive to their environment than are normal children.

"Under the circumstances," says Jacob in evaluating the Chilean study, "the Chilean doctors did as 'scientific' a study as was possible. They didn't have much money to work with, and didn't have the sophisticated monitoring and diagnostic equipment that we have here in the United States. But they were highly experienced specialists and careful observers. They were very careful to diminish as much as one can the effect of environmental differences in the children," he explains. "They did their best to secure as homogeneous a group as they could, which means that the general health of all the children involved was about the same. No, it wasn't your classic double-blind study, but I disagree with anyone who questions its validity."

The study itself was conducted in a fairly standard

manner. Fifty-five children with Down's syndrome were divided into two groups; one group received injections of DMSO with the three amino acids. The second group received no treatment. Other than the injections, both groups of children were given the same frequent and in-depth examinations. "We thought about placebos," reported Dr. Manuel Aspillaga, of the Calvo Mackenna Children's Hospital's Department of Genetics, after the study was published, "but we felt the odor of the DMSO in the treated children would ruin the placebo effect, anyway."

Both groups of children—the DMSO-amino acid group and the control group—were themselves divided into two groups: those between three-and-a-half years and fourteen years old, and those under three-and-a-half years. The rationale behind this grouping was to test yet another hypothesis in the study: that the effects of the therapy would be more pronounced among the younger children, who were still in a relatively early stage of neuronal development. In any case, all the children were given a battery of neurological, psychological and developmental tests at various times during the clinical study. In addition, they received physical examinations. To calculate the development of the children younger than three-and-a-half years old, the doctors used a standard scale—one originally developed by eminent child development specialist Arnold Gesell. A number of standard intelligent quotient tests were used to measure the progress of the older children. In addition, photographs were taken of all the children before, during and after the treatment period to see if there were noticeable changes in the physical features of any of the children.

The study took several months, and in the minds of the specialists who conducted it, it produced very promising results. Improvement was particularly noticeable among the younger children, who showed a greater receptivity to outside stimuli, said the researchers. "This, in turn, pro-voked greater activity and improved muscular tone," they added. The younger children who were treated with DMSO and amino acids also showed what the doctors de-scribed as a "notable increase in their adaptive and social phases over what would usually be expected"—although, said the investigators, the children's language remained almost stationary until a more advanced age.

The results among the older children were also encour-aging. The investigators noted "graphic improvement" in the drawing ability of the treated group. There was no-ticeable improvement in the language and vocabulary of the treated group that didn't show up in the control group. But perhaps the most significant finding is that while the intelligence quotient (I.Q.) of the control group, on average, went from 34 at the beginning of the study to 33 at the end, the I.Q. of the treated group went up from an average of 29 to an average of 40, with none of the children in the treated group dropping in score and 10 showing I.Q. increases of more than 10 points. To be sure, an I.Q. of 40 isn't going to have a measurable impact on a Down's syndrome child's ability to make his way in the world, but it could well mean the difference between being the loving but essentially helpless child Billy King was prior to his starting DMSO-amino acid therapy, and the infinitely more self-sufficient Billy King ten years later.

Can the DMSO-amino acid drug therapy increase I.Q.?

"We really can't answer that question right now," says Stanley Jacob. "We're not even sure of how valid I.Q. tests are when it comes to measuring the development of Down's syndrome children. All we can say is that in this particular study, a group of children who were on the DMSO-amino acid therapy improved and had no seri-ous side effects. However, nontreated children did not improve."

Shortly after the Chilean doctors published their results,

Jacob, with three special-education experts from the University of Oregon, set up his own study similar in some respects to the Chilean study but involving the use of DMSO alone. Sixty-seven mentally retarded children between the ages of four and seventeen were involved initially, but only thirty-nine were studied throughout the duration of the test period.

"We did our best in this study to meet the 'double blind' requirement and to rule out any criteria other than DMSO that might have affected the subjects," explains Jacob. "When the time came to separate the subjects into 'high-dose' and 'low-dose' groups, we brought in an outsider who had no prior knowledge and no subsequent involvement with the study to make the random groupings. None of the project observers, evaluators or members of the staff at the school where the tests were carried out had any knowledge of which children were in which group," he points out. "The only thing lacking was a true placebo group, so what we tried to do was to give a very low dosage to the low-dose group—low enough to produce an odor similar to the other strength DMSO without having any other effects."

This study was designed to see whether DMSO alone could produce changes in language, motor and social behaviors in mentally retarded children, and depending on the way you look at it, it was something of a success and something of a failure. "When you take all the data we were collecting in this study," wrote Jeanne Gabourie, a special-education expert who conducted the study along with Janis W. Becker and Barbara Bateman, "and you view it in terms of the number of measures we were using to see what each child gained or lost there is a definite pattern: the children who received the high-dose DMSO show the most gains, the low-dose children show intermediate gains and the students we observed who didn't take part in the study showed no gains."

Even so, Stanley Jacob wasn't overly pleased with the study. "It was not anybody's fault," he says. "We were trying to quantify, with computers, certain behavioral patterns that are difficult to quantify. We had no way of computing into our results, for instance, the fact that a child could suddenly tell time. What the study ultimately showed us, in addition to safety, was how difficult it is to set up a model that will give you precise data in a condition as individualistic and as unpredictable as retardation."

There has been yet another study, albeit a limited one, done by two Argentinian mental retardation specialists, Ana Giller, of the Pirovano Hospital in Buenos Aires, and Maria E. M. de Bernadou, of the Laboratory of Genetics National Department of Student Health in Buenos Aires. Their study (*Biological Actions of DMSO*, New York Academy of Sciences, 1975, eds. Stanley W. Jacob and Robert Herschler) involved six boys and seven girls between the ages of seven and twenty years, all of whom received DMSO-amino acid therapy over a six-month period, and a control group made up of thirteen mentally retarded children who received what is described as "conventional treatment" and served as a control group. None of the children in this study, however, were Down's syndrome victims; with I.Q.'s ranging from 44 to 80, these were children who are generally characterized as being oligophrenic, which means, simply, being mentally deficient because of faulty development.

In general, the results were positive. The DMSO-amino acid group showed significantly more development in the twelve areas tested—areas including hand-eye coordination, posture and language.

The promising results of early studies such as those described here seemed to have had little impact on mental retardation research in the United States—even though in the early 1970's the FDA seemed sufficiently impressed with the results to dispatch a delegation to Chile

—a fact-finding mission "to evaluate the claimed effectiveness and safety of DMSO used in Chile" not just for mentally retarded children but for a variety of pathological conditions. In the delegation were Dr. Felix de la Cruz, a physician who at the time was the special assistant for pediatrics in the National Institute of Child Health and Human Development; Stanley Jacob, M.D.; and Dr. Frederick Grigsby, a physician who was the acting director of the Division of Surgical and Dental Drug products of the office of Scientific Evaluation in the Bureau of Drugs, U.S. Food and Drug Administration.

The official report on the delegation's findings, written by Dr. Grigsby and submitted to the FDA in 1972, questioned the protocol in the Chilean studies. But it also acknowledged that many of the patients who had been given DMSO and amino acids had indeed shown "clinical improvement," and that this improvement "may in part be due to the effects of DMSO." (Dr. Grigsby noted in the same report that DMSO had produced "promising" results in studies using DMSO-drug combinations in cerebral vascular accidents, leg ulcers, Hodgkin's disease, and Ewing's sarcoma, a rare form of cancer.)

Dr. Grigsby concluded his report to the FDA with a number of specific recommendations. He cautioned that not enough research had yet been presented to establish the safety of DMSO injections, but urged that preclinical animal studies be conducted to determine the relationship of DMSO and the absorption, by the central nervous system, of amino acids. He recommended that the FDA "initiate and become intimately involved in clinical studies —i.e., in the development of protocols and in determining the area of primary interest." So Grigsby, like others who had been to Chile, wasn't sure what to make of the Chilean studies, but he saw enough to realize that something was happening in Chile that could be medically important.

Dr. Grigsby's report worked its way through the creaky

FDA bureaucratic machinery and eventually found its way in the National Institute of Child Health and Human Development Mental Retardation Research Committee. On August 4, 1977, the Institute commenced a two-day meeting, at which time some of the recommendations of the Grigsby report were discussed. The committee voted unanimously to grant a contract that, for starters, would get some animal studies going. Months later, however, another committee somewhere in the government's health bureaucracy vetoed the Institute committee's action. Consequently, nothing has been done in the United States to test the validity of the Chilean study findings, even though Nicholas Weinstein offered to cooperate with American health officials in any way he could to develop protocols and conduct tests that would meet certain scientific criteria and, at the same time, see whether a therapy concept like Merinex held out any hope for mentally retarded children.

Is there a future for DMSO in the treatment of mentally retarded children? Like so many questions surrounding DMSO, it is impossible to give an answer here without tacking on dozens of qualifiers. Nobody, least of all Stanley Jacob, is saying that DMSO can help make mentally retarded children "normal." And it is Jacob's guess that DMSO's ultimate benefit to mental retardation treatment will, in the long run, be as a carrier of substances that normally couldn't pass the blood-brain barrier. "What we have," Jacob says, "are several studies that show promise. We need to do more studies. From what we've seen so far, my feeling is that DMSO, as a therapy unto itself or as a carrier for other substances, has some potential for enhancing the development of mentally retarded children, but it's a long procedure, and you can't expect to see results right away. I don't know the mechanism. Maybe it's nothing more than the fact that DMSO, in a very generalized way, helps the systems of these children work better," he explains. "But I don't know of any development that showed any *more* promise, and the fact that no one is doing any studies in the U.S. in this area is very sad."

Jacob's conservative position notwithstanding, there are nonetheless a number of case studies, in addition to that of Billy King, suggesting that DMSO could at least play an important *role* in helping Down's syndrome children become more functional human beings. One of Jacob's patients, Melody Clark, is nine years old, and has been taking DMSO regularly since she was eleven months old. She'd been diagnosed as a Down's syndrome child five months before she began the therapy. She couldn't stand because her legs, as her mother describes, were like those of "rag dolls." She couldn't roll from her back to her stomach. She couldn't see because her eyes couldn't focus.

"Melody runs, jumps rope, turns somersaults and plays on a trampoline," her mother, Mrs. Dale Clark, now reports. "She is on a second level in reading and excels in math. She is also quite popular with her classmates—very social-minded."

For the record, Melody Clark has worked her way up from a class for "trainables" to a special-education class. She attends Sunday school with normal children. She goes to summer camp. Her dentist, Dr. David K. Preibe, of Wenatchee, Washington, notes that the physical characteristics of Melody's mouth are significantly more "normal" in every aspect compared with those of other Down's syndrome children of similar age. He says that Melody handles the stress of dental treatment as well as children without Down's syndrome. Melody's teacher, Rose M. Mullan, of Wenatchee, Washington, documents what Melody's mother says of the young girl's school work. "She participates in classroom games, shares classroom responsibilities, is conscientious about her school assignments and proud of her academic accomplishments."

How do we know that Melody Clark wouldn't be the

same way without DMSO? We don't, but her mother gives DMSO the credit. "All I know," she says, "is what I've seen with my own eyes. After eight years of being on DMSO, Melody has progressed from a severely retarded child to one who is only mildly retarded. She was born with an extremely high roof in her mouth, and now it is within normal range. I think the progress is because of DMSO. I think it offers parents like us a lot of hope."

CHAPTER VIII

=====================

The Many Faces of DMSO

In 1965, a New Castle, Pennsylvania, woman named Arkie Barlet began experiencing a series of unusual symptoms. She found that she grew tired more easily than before and was having more trouble breathing. She began to notice, too, slight changes in her skin. It was becoming swollen, more leathery and dryer. She went to a doctor, was examined and was told she had a disease she'd never even heard of. The disease was called scleroderma.

Scleroderma, as Arkie Barlet would soon learn, is a punishing disease of unknown origin whose painful and disfiguring symptoms result from an abnormal build-up in the system of the fibrous protein substance known as collagen. The swelling, leatheriness, increased denseness and hardness of the skin are among the effects of this collagen build-up. "Your skin," Arkie describes, "becomes impermeable and very tight. You're tired a lot of the time—even when you wake up in the morning. Your fingers get very sensitive to the cold. You get calcium deposits in your

joints and you have trouble bending. Scleroderma even affects the saliva in your mouth and the tear ducts in your
eyes," she explains, adding that "some people walk around
all the time with a gagging sensation."

To learn that you have a disease for which there is no
known effective treatment is bad enough. But to know of
nobody who is suffering what you are going through is
worse. So Arkie Barlet did a remarkable thing. She sat
down and began composing letters to newspapers
throughout the country. She wanted other people who
also had scleroderma to get in touch with her. Fighting
the constant pain in her gnarled fingers, she wrote more
than 2,000 letters, nearly all of which were published, and
she says she will never forgive two papers—one in Can-
ton, Ohio, and the other *The New York Times*—for not
printing the letter unless she paid for it. "As if," Arkie
says, "I was trying to sell a product."

Soon she began receiving letters from all over the country, many of which came from people who felt the same
need as Arkie felt: to communicate with somebody who
was going through what they were going through. She
wrote letters back, she had phone conversations with people throughout the country, and the upshot of it all is
something called the Scleroderma International Foundation, whose headquarters are in Arkie Barlet's New Castle
home. "We write each other," says Arkie. "We phone one
another. We distribute information. And once a year about
200 people who have scleroderma come from all over the
country and we have a big get-together at a local hotel.
Some of the people don't have any fingers or legs because
this disease can cause gangrene-like conditions, but we
don't feel sorry for ourselves. Whenever I talk to the people we hire as speakers, I have to remind them that we're
not looking for people to feel sorry for us. We want to
laugh and enjoy ourselves."

Arkie Barlet believes that if it weren't for DMSO she,

too, might be an amputee or could well be dead by now. She uses specially formulated DMSO every day, rubbing it all over her body. "It cuts the pain," she says. "It makes my skin a little softer. It lets me live a reasonably normal life. I have a job. I'm as productive as any employee I work with even though I still have a problem with my fingers. When I come home at night, I have enough energy to take care of my father, to answer letters and to talk to people on the phone."

Arkie Barlet isn't going to tell you that DMSO has "cured" her of scleroderma. But it relieves some of the symptoms. It helps make life a little more bearable for her. And there are thousands upon thousands of people throughout the United States, not all scleroderma victims, but people with a variety of illnesses who may not know how DMSO works but do know one thing: it makes them feel better, it brings them relief.

"DMSO is not a miracle panacea," Stanley Jacob says. "We never said it was. All we've been saying all along is that here is a compound that does a lot of interesting things—a compound that is safe and a compound that's abundant enough so that anybody can afford it. Most of all, it's a compound that brings a lot of people relief that they can't get from any other medication."

Exactly *how* many different conditions DMSO can help is difficult to say, given the fact that it relieves so many different conditions and diseases. Here, in any event, is a partial list of the conditions in which DMSO, either by itself or in conjunction with other drugs, has helped to bring relief to some or most of the symptoms.

Burns

Its ability to provide prompt and dramatic relief of the pain that comes with burns, and to prevent some of the blistering that frequently occurs, was one of the first medical properties discovered about DMSO. DMSO is so useful a burn agent, in fact, that Dr. J. Harold Brown, of Seattle, keeps a bottle of it on hand in the kitchen of his home. As Dr. Brown and others familiar with DMSO point out, the sooner you use DMSO on a burn, the better the chances of cutting the pain and minimizing the scarring.

Stanley Jacob treats minor first- and second-degree thermal burns by running the burned area under cold water and then immediately applying anywhere from a 50 percent to a 70 percent DMSO solution, using it as often as necessary, for three days, to keep the pain down. "The more you use," he says, "the better." With third-degree burn patients, he uses DMSO with local antibiotics and other conventional burn treatments.

Although no clinical tests on humans have ever been conducted that would measure the true effectiveness of DMSO on burns, there is reason to believe from animal studies and some clinical reports that if you put DMSO on a burn quickly enough, skin that would normally die and fall off can be saved. "The skin doesn't always die immediately with a burn," says Jacob. "DMSO seems to protect skin that would otherwise die, and most patients do not develop blister formations."

Bursitis

Bursitis, an inflammatory condition affecting the bursa —a fluid-containing sac, made of connective tissue, that encloses the joints and reduces their friction when they move—responds well to topical DMSO treatment, although more so in acute cases than in chronic conditions. Arthur Steinberg, in his report at the 1966 New York Academy of Sciences symposium on DMSO reported favorable response with eight of nine chronic bursitis patients that he treated topically with DMSO. The German physicians John and Laudahn reported a complete remission of symptoms in about 78 percent. Their success rate in treating chronic bursitis patients over a three-month period was roughly the same, although there was a higher percentage of failures. Stanley Jacob's clinical experiences with DMSO and bursitis indicate that topical DMSO is effective about 80 percent of the time with acute bursitis. Chronic conditions, he reports, are somewhat more resistant. After reviewing the literature, the National Academy of Sciences described DMSO as being "as efficacious as currently accepted methods of treatment in acute painful shoulder of other than traumatic origin."

Arthritis

As already described in chapter V, DMSO in various dosages has been shown in several clinical studies to be effective against the pain and inflammation in many of the more than 100 different forms of arthritis, and, in certain rheumatoid arthritis patients, to bring about a stabilization of the disease. Generally speaking, DMSO is more effective in relieving the acute pain in osteoarthritis and rheumatoid arthritis than the chronic pain in both of these conditions, and—as noted in chapter V—patients with arthritic conditions above the waist have responded better than patients with arthritic conditions below the waist, and arthritic fingers and hands therefore generally respond to the pain-relieving properties of DMSO better than arthritic hips and knees.

Although there is no evidence that DMSO has any effect on the underlying causes of arthritis (whatever they may be), there is evidence to suggest that rheumatoid arthritis patients who take a carefully supervised DMSO program experience a noticeable stabilization of the condition. And in many patients, although topical DMSO is only partially effective in relieving pain and increasing joint mobility, injections of DMSO are often quite effective. Stanley Jacob sees DMSO not as the ultimate arthritis medication but as a very useful adjunct to other drugs. One of the best features of DMSO as an arthritis medication is that it relieves pain without causing the troublesome side effects that other commonly prescribed medications produce.

Cancer

There is no evidence to suggest that DMSO is an effective cancer treatment *per se*, but a growing amount of evidence suggests that DMSO, in combination with other cancer drugs, should play an important role in chemotherapy in the future. Drs. Jorge Cornejo Garrido and Raul Escobar Lagos, of the Military Hospital in Santiago, Chile, reported at the 1975 New York Academy of Sciences symposium on DMSO that a combination of DMSO and the drug cyclophosphamide produced promising results in a majority of sixty-five patients diagnosed as having incurable malignancies. Cyclophosphamide is a powerful chemical known to have anti-cancer properties, but it is also highly toxic, producing nausea and anemia. The Chilean doctors found that when mixed with DMSO, the cyclophosphamide not only became less toxic but was potentiated as well. The doctors reported the best success with patients suffering from lymphomas, and were also able to produce either objective or subjective remissions in twenty-three of twenty-six post-mastectomy patients. All but two of the mastectomy patients tolerated the treatment with a minimum of side effects. Approximately one third of the patients in the study died or saw their conditions worsening throughout the six-month treatment period, but many of them had experienced remissions lasting more than a year.

Back Pain

Most chronic back-pain patients who have been treated with DMSO at Stanley Jacob's clinic have experienced relief that other pain medications were unable to deliver. Several patients with pain resulting from pressure on the sciatic nerve have experienced relief through topical administration of DMSO only, but others have required DMSO injections as well. Relief in many chronic pain conditions doesn't become noticeable until at least six or eight weeks after a patient is first treated with DMSO.

Chronic Pain

A number of chronic pain conditions for which conventional treatment fails to bring relief respond to DMSO treatment, including pain resulting from pressure on the sciatic nerve, "phantom limb" pain in amputees, and various kinds of arthritic pain. But relief sometimes takes several weeks and may require DMSO injections in addition to topical treatments. "Pain is such an individual phenomenon," says Jacob, "that you have to deal with each patient on a separate basis. You have to vary treatment, depending on the kind of pain, where the pain is located, and how long the patient has been suffering from it."

"Frozen Shoulder"

Most clinical reports indicate that DMSO in a 70 percent solution applied topically will restore movement and relieve pain in the majority of frozen shoulder patients, although the number of treatments necessary to produce relief can range from five or six to more than two dozen. Generally, but not always, the patients who are going to respond well to the treatment begin to notice some measure of relief after the first or second application of DMSO.

Interstitial Cystitis

Interstitial cystitis was, as of the spring of 1981, the only condition for which a DMSO medication is approved by the Food and Drug Administration. It is a very painful and uncontrollable bladder condition caused by inflammation in the lining of the bladder. The FDA granted approval to DMSO for this condition on the basis of clinical studies showing that 64 percent of male interstitial cystitis patients and 54 percent of female patients experienced "significant symptomatic relief with it." DMSO doesn't cure the underlying cause of the disease, which is unknown, but is the only substance thus far that has been able to ease the pain and the irritation that are characteristic of interstitial cystitis.

Scleroderma

Clinical studies from the Cleveland Clinic show that DMSO is more effective than any other medication now available in its ability to promote the healing of fingertip and toe ulcers—one of the many symptoms of scleroderma that are caused by an abnormal build-up of collagen in the tissues. Patients taking part in studies being supervised by Dr. Arthur Scherbel of the Cleveland Clinic report in many instances not only healing but much less pain and a softening of the skin tissue. Scleroderma patients who have the ulcers of the disease are sometimes faced with the need for amputation, since the ulcers often lead to gangrene-like conditions in the fingers and toes.

Dental Pain

Since the late 1960's, Dr. Robert L. Anderson, a Portland dentist who specializes in restorative work, has been using DMSO to solve the problem some patients have with hypersensitive teeth that cause pain after extensive restorative work has been done. The cause of this pain is something known as intrapulpal inflammation, which is inflammation that results from trauma caused by the dental work itself. Dr. Anderson has found that when cotton doused with a 100 percent DMSO solution is applied for ten to twenty minutes after any extensive work has been done on a tooth, the inflammation recedes almost immediately. DMSO, he says, has virtually eliminated postoperative dental pain, even among patients who have undergone a full day of restorative dental work.

Ear Diseases

There are a number of ear conditions in which DMSO is quite effective. The inflammatory ear condition known as funicular otitis responds to a combination of 90 percent DMSO and the antibiotics Terramycin and erythromycin, according to a clinical report by Hans Asen (Biological Actions of DMSO, New York Academy of Sciences, Vol. 141, 1967, ed. Edward M. Weyer). Washington physician J. Harold Brown reports good success by treating the condition known as aerotitis—a painful earache that some people suffer when they fly—by spraying DMSO into the nose. Other ear specialists have found topical DMSO with a local anesthetic useful when draining middle-ear infections. Normally these operations require general anesthetics.

Eye Diseases

Since 1973, a Longview, Washington, ophthalmologist named Robert V. Hill has been using DMSO for a number of difficult-to-treat retinal diseases, among them diabetic retinopathy, macular degeneration and retinitis pigmentosa. Interestingly enough, he began these studies as the result of reports from patients who were taking DMSO for musculoskeletal disorders and who were reporting that their vision improved. In one study, Hill treated fifty-one patients with one of two types of retinal disorder and found that twenty-three of them were able to see more clearly, and nine showed improved visual fields and five reported improvement in adapting to the dark. His treatment procedure in each was to apply a 50 percent DMSO solution directly to the cornea of the eye by immersing the eye in an eye-cup for thirty seconds, twice daily. As of this writing, he is completing a new phase in the study to determine whether the subjective improvement reported by patients can be replicated in a more controlled experimental protocol. "The preliminary evidence gives us reason for cautious optimism," he says. "Toxicity appears to be minimal. Controlled studies seem necessary in the area of eye diseases."

Gastrointestinal Diseases

There is experimental evidence in rats to suggest that DMSO, by reducing the secretion of stomach acids, can promote the healing of ulcers. But there is amost no clinical evidence in the United States to indicate how applicable this finding is to humans. A French company now holds a patent on an oral DMSO medicine that is said to help relieve some of the inflammation of ileitis and colitis, and some DMSO patients who suffer from gastrointestinal inflammations report relief from these problems after taking DMSO for other conditions. "We still know very little about the effect of DMSO on the gastrointestinal tract," says Stanley Jacob. "It's much too early to tell what therapeutic benefit DMSO is going to have in any of these conditions."

Headaches

Headaches rooted in muscle tension or sinusitis respond well to topical DMSO treatment. One application directly on the area of pain can bring relief lasting four to six hours. Migraine and cluster headaches are not as predictable, and most studies show that DMSO is not particularly effective as a pain-relieving agent in these kinds of headaches. The probable reason for this is that DMSO's vasodilating properties expand blood vessels whose pressure against the cranial cavity may be responsible for such headaches in the first place. Among the several clinical studies done on DMSO and its effect on headaches is one conducted by Drs. Lester S. Blumenthal and Marvin

Fuchs, at the Headache Clinic of the George Washington University Hospital in Washington, D.C. They reported their findings at the 1966 New York Academy of Sciences symposium on DMSO, stating that they were able to bring "good to excellent" results in 80 percent of the patients who came to them with muscle tension headaches, and 100 percent of patients with sinus headaches. With migraine and cluster headaches "good to excellent" results were reported in only one-third of the cases.

Gout

Gout is a very painful but not life-threatening or necessarily crippling form of arthritis that occurs because of an abnormal build-up of uric acid. The German physicians Heinz John and Gerhard Laudahn (Biological Actions of DMSO, New York Academy of Sciences, Vol. 141, 1967, ed. Chauncey D. Leake) reported a complete remission of symptoms in sixteen of nineteen gouty arthritis patients they treated. Stanley Jacob reports a 75 to 80 percent success rate with topical DMSO in gout.

Hemorrhoids

There have been no clinical studies in the United States that would show how well DMSO compares to other hemorrhoid remedies currently on the market, but a new solution in Germany, of DMSO mixed with enzymes and vitamin A, is generally superior to any topical hemorrhoidal ointment now available.

Herpes Virus Infections

Some—but not all—herpes conditions respond well to DMSO treatment; the most responsive is herpes simplex (fever blister). Although DMSO by itself and applied topically can bring relief to these conditions most of the time, a more effective way of treating herpes zoster is with a mixture of DMSO and the drug idoxuridine (IDU) —a prescriptive mixture that has been approved for use in Great Britain.

Infections

DMSO as an infection fighter is best used in combinations, and one of the best combinations is a mixture of DMSO with iodine. This combination is particularly effective for deep-seated infections. Research indicates that many DMSO combinations are effective in a variety of skin infections.

Peyronie's Disease

Peyronie's disease is a condition in which plaque builds up in the penis, producing extreme pain whenever a patient gets an erection. Peyronie's disease patients at the DMSO clinic in Portland receive topical application of DMSO directly in the penis, and Stanley Jacob reports relief in about 50 percent of the cases he treats. "We're not seeing rapid, significant improvement in curvature but the newer DMSO preparations we are employing are superior to DMSO water." In one of the few studies on DMSO and Peyronie's disease, two Cleveland urologists, Lester Persky and Bruce H. Stewart, reported that of thirteen men with the condition who were treated, six were improved enough to resume reasonably normal intercourse, and one patient showed a complete disappearance of the plaque caused by the disease. (Biological Actions of DMSO, New York Academy of Sciences: Vol. 141, 1967, ed. Chauncey D. Leake).

Phlebitis

DMSO's potential in phlebitis and other related vascular disorders lies mainly in its combined use with other drugs; such combinations are now prescriptive in Europe and Asia. Stanley Jacob's clinical experience with phlebitis patients in Portland shows that when topically applied, DMSO relieves some of the superficial clotting symptomatic of thrombophlebitis.

Pruritus Ani

Pruritus ani is an extremely uncomfortable itching condition that often produces infection and extreme pain during defecation. Limited reports show a 90 percent success rate in treatment of the condition with a 70 percent DMSO solution applied directly to the itching areas.

Raynaud's Disease

Patients who suffer from Raynaud's disease experience painful spasms of their fingers and toes whenever these extremities come into contact with cold. Stanley Jacob's success rate in treating this condition with DMSO alone is about 50 percent. "It doesn't attack the root of the problem," he says, "which is a lack of circulation in the extremities, but it produces temporary vasodilation—more blood flow—and provides symptomatic relief."

Shingles

In shingles, technically known as herpes zoster, blisters form and erupt in various parts of the body, causing searing pain. The disease has a neurological component, so that in some cases, even after the blisters have healed, the pain persists. Early clinical work in the 1960's showed that DMSO, as a primary agent, could ease much of the pain that shingles produces, but a more effective treatment—one that is prescriptive in Great Britain—is a combination of DMSO with the anti-viral substance idoxuridine. By itself, idoxuridine (IDU) can inhibit the growth of the herpes zoster virus, but its effectiveness increases when a 5 percent IDU solution is mixed with 100 percent DMSO solution. In 1970, a controlled study by a team of British physicians showed that the mixture of IDU and DMSO could not only relieve the pain of shingles when used on a short-term basis, but could accelerate healing when used continuously. Patients for whom IDU and DMSO is prescribed apply the mixture directly to their lesions. The 1970 study described two methods of application, the first employing a paintbrush to apply the substance four times a day to each affected area of the body, a second calling for saturating a gauze pad cut to cover the affected area, and then moistening the pad daily for four days with the solution.

Stanley Jacob, in his Portland clinic, has treated a handful of shingles patients for post-herpetic pain (the pain that lingers after the lesions have healed). He reports success in three patients who have had this pain for more than two years.

Sinusitis

A specially formulated 50 percent DMSO nose-drop medication is producing what Stanley Jacob describes as "excellent results" among the sinusitis patients he treats in Portland. The drops give a brief stinging sensation, but clear the nasal passages in less than thirty seconds. One big advantage DMSO has over other nose drops and nose sprays, points out Jacob, is that as time goes on, people require less and less of the DMSO to clear their sinuses. This is an interesting pattern that DMSO achieves in many conditions, and in this respect, DMSO differs from other medications whose dosages must be gradually increased as patients develop tolerance.

Tendinitis

The inflammation of the tendon known as tendinitis—like most sofe-tissue inflammations—responds well to topically applied DMSO in strengths in excess of 60 percent. As in bursitis, acute conditions respond more favorably and in a shorter period of time than chronic conditions. Heinz John and Gerhard Laudahn's research shows that nearly 60 percent of the patients treated with DMSO for tendinitis, as well as two similar conditions—periostitis and epicondylitus (tennis elbow)—experienced noticeable relief of pain in two to three weeks. They also reported in their 1965 study only 60 failures among 409 cases of these conditions. Stanley Jacob describes his clinical experiences with various types of tendinitis as being good but unpredictable. "A lot depends on where the condition is. We're more successful with tendinitis above the waist than below the waist."

DMSO in Veterinary Medicine

If horses could speak, there would probably be as many testimonies to the effectiveness of DMSO in the equine world as there are today among humans. DMSO has been approved for veterinary use in 90 percent gel form since 1970, and a U.S. House of Representatives Select Committee on Aging questionnaire sent to a random sampling of veterinarians in 1980 revealed that 70 percent of the veterinarians in the United States use DMSO in their practice, with 90 percent of this number considering it effective in reducing inflammation, pain and other arthritic symptoms in animals. Interestingly, too, 80 percent of the veterinarians who responded to the questionnaire felt that, on the basis of their experience with DMSO in animals, the substance would be safe and effective for humans.

DMSO is now approved by the FDA for treatment in the following, to name only some conditions: contusions, sprains, cuts, excess scar tissue, postoperative infections, myositis, rattlesnake bite—even torn toenails. And its anti-inflammatory effect on conditions in animals similar to conditions in humans is well documented. One Portland, Oregon, veterinarian maintains that DMSO is every bit as powerful in its anti-inflammatory properties as corticosteroids and butazolidin—and without the side effects. (Yes, animals suffer side effects from medication, too.) "It reduces the time required for wound healing by one-third," he says. "When I combine it with various antiseptics, it carries these agents deeper into contaminated areas. I use it intravenously in shock and concussion, and its effect is dramatic and lasting." A Topeka, Kansas, veterinarian who uses DMSO for his own tennis elbow says he can't understand why the drug has been "so slow to hit the human field." An Absecon, New Jersey, vet says that while DMSO is not a panacea, it's certainly effective. "What I like about it," he says, "is that it's an excellent vehicle for getting other anti-inflammatory drugs into a joint without tapping the joint cavity and without risking infection."

Dozens of laboratory studies back up these endorsements. Two of the first research veterinarians to work with DMSO were M. B. Tiegland and V. R. Saurino, who reported their findings at the 1966 New York Academy of Sciences DMSO symposium. Horses that are hypersensitized with purified fractions of human gamma globulin develop a massive inflammatory reaction that prevents the animals from moving their necks. Drs. Tiegland and Saurino compared the anti-inflammatory effects of DMSO on such horses with conventional treatment, and found DMSO to be vastly superior. The two veterinarians also treated twenty-two cases of tendinitis and reported results "superior to that produced with any previously used external treatment." Other reports, both in the literature and privately from veterinarians, show that DMSO can reduce the swelling and sensitivity that often occur after an animal has been tightly bandaged, can control excess granulation of tissue in open wounds, and can promote the healing of lesions.

What DMSO can do for horses, it can also do for dogs. Robert P. Knowles, who conducted studies at the University of Miami School of Medicine and reported his findings at the 1966 DMSO symposium in New York, found that DMSO was effective in a number of dog illnesses and conditions. He treated nine dogs with severe dermatitis, using a combination of DMSO, nitrofurazone and nystatin, and brought about recovery in eight of the dogs and improvement in the other. He treated eight cases of an inflammation that frequently occurs as the result of vaccine use in dogs, and was able to bring down the swelling and reduce the inflammation in one week. He treated twenty dogs and cats that were having allergic reactions to flea bites and reported complete success in each instance.

One of Dr. Knowles's most interesting cases involved a racing greyhound that had sustained severe tendinitis in one paw. "Generally," he points out, "this type of injury will eliminate a dog from competition permanently or drop him one or two grades on the competitive scale. It is rare for a dog to recover from this kind of injury and still retain his former speed."

Knowles began treating the dog two months after it first suffered the injury. There was swelling and tenderness, and an X-ray showed that the tendon was enlarged. "We began applying 90 percent DMSO three times a day," Knowles reports. "The swelling was reduced noticeably in three days, and after one week, there was only a slight palpable difference between the affected tendon and its companion on the unaffected leg."

In its first race, after two months, the greyhound developed lameness, tenderness and swelling in the affected tendon. This time Knowles gave him DMSO immediately, and the pain and swelling promptly disappeared.

"We kept up the treatment for 30 days and rested the animal an additional 90 days," he explains. Once back at its former grade, the dog continued to race without lameness. "Within nine months of our initial examination," Knowles reports, "the dog had established two new track records."

At least one man who isn't surprised at this story is Robert Herschler, whose black Labrador has twice had a brush with death and has twice pulled through, in Herschler's judgment, because of DMSO. "In 1962," Herschler says, "the dog was hit by a motorcycle and he made history. He became the first animal intentionally treated with DMSO for serious trauma." Two years later, while Herschler and the dog were hunting pheasants, a rattlesnake bit the dog in the head. The dog not only survived but after two hours rest was once again fetching pheasants. "Maybe he was just a tough dog," Herschler says. "But maybe it was the fact that as soon as he was bit, I saturated his head and shoulders with DMSO."

The most intriguing animal studies with DMSO have been done recently by a Washington state veterinarian named Jack Metcalf, who has been working with dummy foals—newborn horses whose immature brain development so retards the horse's behavior that it doesn't even know how to nurse. Metcalf has shown that intravenous treatments of DMSO three times daily not only can get the foals to begin nursing, but serve to enhance and accelerate their overall development. "What's exciting about Metcalf's work," says Stanley Jacob, "is that the dummy foal is the only natural animal model we have evaluated for retardation. The significance to humans can't be overlooked and should be investigated."

DMSO in Agriculture

It was Robert Herschler's 1959 discovery that some plant fungicides penetrated much more quickly and deeply into plant tubers and trees after being mixed with DMSO that originally tweaked his interest in the chemical as a therapeutic substance in humans. However, DMSO has shown itself through the years to be as varied in its beneficial effects on plants as it is in humans. Here are some things it can do.

1. It enhances the ability of plant roots to absorb nutrients, water and pesticides.

2. It gives both plants and vegetables grown in a greenhouse much the same color—and in the case of vegetables, taste—as that of field-grown plants and vegetables.

3. It stimulates plant, flower and vegetable growth.

4. It protects plants and vegetables from freezing.

5. It helps prevent disease in many plants, trees and vegetables.

Numerous studies support these properties. Robert L. Weintraub, who wrote the agricultural chapter in *The Basic Concepts of DMSO* (Marcel Dekker, Inc., New York, 1971), cites studies in which shoots of zinnia, marigold, bean, corn and cucumber given regular "fixes" of DMSO grew taller than control shoots of the same plants. He also cites a study showing that young potato plants sprayed with 0.5 percent DMSO and then kept at a temperature of twenty degrees Fahrenheit for four hours suffer some degree of injury, but not nearly as much as young potato plants sprayed only with water. "The DMSO-treated plants," Weintraub reports, "were larger, grew more vigorously and produced the equivalent of 100 sacks per acre more tubers than the water-treated controls." He also gives credence to a theory now being advanced by some botanists that DMSO may well be a natural constituent of certain plants. Both of DMSO's metabolites—dimethylsulfide and dimethylsulfone—have been identified in various plant species; and while there is no evidence that DMSO can be oxidized to dimethylsulfone in plant tissue, the presence of these metabolites in plants is a further indication of DMSO's low toxicity.

Several other plant studies with DMSO, each reported at the New York Academy of Sciences DMSO symposium in 1966, are worth mention. In one of the studies, by Ralph Garren, Jr., of the Department of Horticulture of Oregon State University, four healthy, uniformly selected strawberry plants were transplanted into separate one-gallon metal cans, each containing the same soil. Two of the plants received a DMSO solution and two received a similar amount of distilled water. After a ninety-six-hour wait, the investigators added radioactively labeled sodium phosphate to each of the four plants. The results showed clearly that the DMSO-treated plants had a greater ability to absorb phosphorus through their root systems.

In a second study, Harry L. Keil of the Crops Research Division of the U.S. Department of Agriculture in Beltsville, Maryland, compared the relative protective power of a number of substances known to inhibit bacterial growth in certain plants and fruits. Keil found that although the drug known as oxytetracycline satisfactorily controlled bacterial spots on peaches, its capacity to control bacteria was enhanced by adding DMSO. As Keil theorized, "Apparently DMSO increases penetration and translocation of the active antibiotic."

In yet another agricultural study reported at the 1966 symposium, Leo A. Sciuchetti showed that DMSO enhances the effects of certain growth regulators—substances that control the growth of plants—used in four species of datura.

"All in all," says Robert Herschler, "what the agricultural studies demonstrate are both effectiveness and safety.

These studies have been carried out by both the U.S. Department of Agriculture and university scientists. The agricultural studies are important in and of themselves but important, too, for what they tell us about DMSO in general."

CHAPTER IX

<hr>

How Safe Is DMSO?

Sitting with about ten other patients in the hallway outside the third-floor DMSO clinic at the University of Oregon Health Sciences Center was a small, delicate woman in her mid-sixties. Three months earlier, she was telling a visitor, her arthritis was so crippling that her husband had to wheel her in. Now, she said, she could walk with the aid of a "walker," and she felt sure that within a few months, she could get by with nothing more than a cane. "Then again," she said, "DMSO could be dangerous. Twenty years from now, when I'm eighty-three, I may find out that I can't have any children."

Can DMSO cause infertility? Is there a chance that it could produce in newborns the horrible deformities that the tranquilizer thalidomide produced? Can DMSO cause cancer? Will your hair fall out if you take too much DMSO? Will taking DMSO cause blindness?

To anybody who has followed the DMSO story closely over the past several years and has read some of the reports the FDA has issued, these questions are not inappropriate. Indeed, every article you read in the lay press about DMSO stresses that its safety has not yet been proven in the long run, and there is frequent mention of animal studies that suggest possible toxic effects in humans. The very fact that after nearly twenty years DMSO has yet to gain the full endorsement of the FDA has helped to create in the public mind a general feeling that whatever its benefits, it may have potentially dangerous long-term side effects.

"I don't blame anybody for being cautious about *any* new substance," says Stanley Jacob, "and this includes DMSO. But we have to look at the record. No drug that I know of has been subjected to more studies designed to determine how safe it is, and the bottom line is: in nearly twenty years, with millions of people using DMSO throughout the world, there has yet to be one well-documented instance of DMSO producing a lethal toxic effect. I've been taking DMSO myself nearly every day since 1963. I've given it to my children. I'm not saying that DMSO doesn't have side effects," he explains. "There is no drug that doesn't have *some* side effects. But the side effects of DMSO are very mild compared to most other drugs—including aspirin. I will match the safety record of DMSO against any therapeutic substance in medicine."

The point about every drug carrying some degree of risk to the person who takes it is worth remembering before examining the "record" Jacob mentions. Everyone acknowledges that whenever you're evaluating the safety of a drug, you must always weigh the potential benefit against the potential risk. If a drug has the potential to cure a normally fatal disease, the fact that it might produce nausea or insomnia or temporary baldness is a small price to pay. On the other hand, you wouldn't take a drug with the same side effects if you were interested in getting relief from, say, athlete's foot.

One of the things that has complicated the question of DMSO's safety is that it has both a therapeutic potential in routine, everyday medical problems, such as sprains, and a therapeutic potential in much more serious, life-threatening conditions. What's more, because it is readily available as an industrial solvent, the possibility of patients abusing DMSO is much greater than would be the case if DMSO were like, for instance, penicillin, in which case the only way you could get it would be through a doctor's prescription. The question of "control" has bothered some FDA officials ever since DMSO first came to their attention in 1963. And it is not unreasonable to suggest that much of what the FDA has done with respect to DMSO since 1963 has been more a reflection of its concern with maintaining control over the use of DMSO than of a genuine desire to determine how safe and effective the substance is.

If DMSO is approved as a general-purpose medication for sprains and aches, it could very well become as commonly used as aspirin. And because DMSO is a relatively easy drug to get, and because people are going to use it topically as you would use suntan lotion or over-the-counter liniment, how are you going to control how frequently people use it and how much they use of it?

In the United States, as in most countries, the task of evaluating the safety of a drug rests in the hands of such government agencies as the Food and Drug Administration.

The law that gave the federal government the right to set standards for the purity, potency and effectiveness of any drugs sold either in the District of Columbia or through interstate commerce was passed by Congress in 1902. The Food and Drug Administration itself, however, was not created until 1927, and it wasn't until eleven years later, after some 100 people died from an elixir including sulfanilamide, that Congress passed the Food, Drug, and

Cosmetic Act—the chief provision of which was that the FDA had to approve a drug as safe before a drug company could market it. This law was toughened considerably in 1962 in the wake of the thalidomide disaster and mandated proof of both safety and effectiveness.

Today, a drug company that wants to market a new substance must first prove to the FDA that the drug is both safe and effective for the condition it is meant to relieve. The FDA itself doesn't normally conduct tests. It merely evaluates data supplied it by researchers or investigators who have been hired by drug companies to conduct studies. Accordingly, a company introducing a new substance sends to the FDA animal or other laboratory studies that describe the drug's pharmacological activities and its potential toxicity. On the basis of this information, the FDA issues or denies something known as an IND, a Notice of a Claimed Investigational Exemption for a New Drug. The IND grants to the drug company permission to conduct limited studies on humans. From this point, there are three phases to the testing procedure, under current FDA regulations. The first phase involves toxicity testing—giving the drug in small amounts and for short periods to human volunteers to see if toxic effects turn up. Phase II is designed to establish the effectiveness of a drug and to get a better fix on its safety. Once phase II is complete, the company must then conduct controlled studies with a larger group of patients—the FDA usually requires data from 1,000 to 3,000 patients—in order to establish that the drug has an acceptable ratio of benefit versus risk. Once these studies are done, the company then submits all the information to the FDA, as part of a New Drug Application—or NDA. It is on the basis of this material that the FDA either grants its approval or asks for additional studies. In the strict sense of the word, the FDA never really *disapproves* an NDA, it simply keeps sending NDA's back for additional data.

There is a noble purpose behind the law that has set up these regulations. Yet even staunch FDA supporters are beginning to concede that the current system is frighteningly expensive, unwieldy and, in many respects, counterproductive. Under the best of conditions, it takes several years before a company completes all three testing phases to the FDA's satisfaction, with the result that before a drug company can market a new drug, it has to be prepared to spend as much as $70 million or more. It's no wonder, then, that most major drug companies in the United States are introducing and developing new drugs abroad. Nor is it any wonder that there are many drugs routinely prescribed in other parts of the world that have yet to be approved in the United States, one of which, of course, is DMSO.

From the beginning, DMSO has been subjected to all the same kinds of safety and effectiveness tests that any drug requiring FDA approval has undergone; but for now, we'll consider only those tests that have been designed to establish its level of toxicity.

Scientists who conduct toxicity studies on new drugs have a none-too-subtle method of gathering information. They pump laboratory animals with doses well beyond what would be the normal dosage range in humans—and then watch to see what happens. They administer the drug in various ways: orally, topically, through the gut, rectally and intravenously. The object in most of these experiments is to see how much of the drug it takes to kill a certain animal. Scientists try to establish something known as the LD_{50}—the amount of the drug, on one-gram-of-drug per one-kilogram-of-animal weight basis, that is sufficient to kill 50 percent of a group of experimental animals. However, even the animals that survive are sacrificed so that scientists can study the effects of a drug on various organs and tissues.

DMSO has been tested along these lines more than any

other experimental drug ever developed. Tests have been done in eleven different animal species, eight more than the FDA requirement. Says Stanley Jacob, with more than a touch of irony in his voice: "DMSO has been responsible for the unnecessary death of more laboratory animals than any other drug in the history of medicine."

The earliest toxicity tests were done on rats. Investigators learned that if you wanted to kill a rat with DMSO, you had to give the rat, orally, from 19.7 to 28.3 grams of it per kilogram of animal. Rats given this much pure alcohol (which, incidentally, is a substance contained in many prescription drugs, not to mention beer, wine and spirits) will have perished long before you reach this level. The LD_{50} level of alcohol in rats—for the record—is about 13.7 grams per kilogram.

This is for DMSO given *orally*, mind you. Practically speaking, it is impossible to hurt yourself seriously with an overdose of DMSO applied topically. This is because the skin can only absorb DMSO at a fixed rate. Anything over this simply drips off. Your only concern would be an allergic reaction that would manifest itself long before the effects would pose any serious threat to your well-being.

According to a Merck, Sharpe and Dohme study submitted to the FDA in 1965, several oral studies in other species of animals suggest that what is true for rats in terms of lethal toxic levels is also true for most animals, the lone exception being the rabbit. Rabbits have a lower LD_{50} level for DMSO than other species—the reason, according to Robert Herschler, being related to DMSO's antimicrobial activity. "The rabbit and some other animals," he suggests, "need certain microorganisms in their digestive systems to assure digestion and assimilation. DMSO probably upsets some of the microflora, but," he explains, "this appears to be a very species-specific phenomenon."

As far as the amount of DMSO that would be lethal to a human being, one must obviously use an indirect ap-

proach. A comparison between DMSO and alcohol is illu-
minating. Alcohol becomes deadly to humans when the
so-called "blood alcohol" level—the amount of alcohol in
milligrams per 100 milliliters of blood, expressed in a percentage—is approximately one-half of one percent. To
achieve this blood level, a person of average weight would
have to consume, within the space of an hour, more than a
quart and a half of eighty-proof vodka, or about twenty-
five cans of beer. (Fortunately, the average person will either have passed out before reaching the lethal dosage
level, or the alcohol will have triggered a vomiting reflex.)

If we use the lethal dosage level for rats as a comparative model, and remember that alcohol is far more toxic
than DMSO, you can figure that before DMSO can kill
you, you'd have to drink at least two quarts within an
hour, which is more than most people who use DMSO
every day get into their systems in two months! Even
then, death is unlikely, for you would trigger the same
reflex action you'd trigger if you ever tried to take more
water into your system than your system could handle.
As Robert Herschler observes, "If you're looking to commit suicide, I don't recommend DMSO."

But what of non-lethal side effects? Here, too, literally
hundreds of studies have been done, not only on animals
but on humans as well, and, except for one effect—
changes in the eye lenses of certain laboratory animals—
no potentially serious toxic effect from DMSO has been
uncovered. What's more, these lens changes, to be discussed in a moment, have yet to show up in humans in the
nearly twenty years that DMSO has been used for medical
purposes. In a National Academy of Sciences Committee
report, submitted to the FDA in 1971, DMSO was described as having a "relatively low toxicity level," apart
from the unexplained eye effects in certain animals. Even
the FDA acknowledges today that the safety of DMSO on
a short-term basis is no longer a matter of concern.

But the FDA didn't always talk this way. Indeed, it has only been since 1980 that the FDA removed from DMSO several restrictive conditions covering human testing procedures. One of the studies that forced the FDA to change its policies with respect to DMSO testing (although it has taken nearly thirteen years) was done in 1967, fourteen months after the FDA ordered its ban on clinical testing of the substance.

The study was designed and carried out by Dr. Frank Hull, a practicing ophthalmologist, and was published in the *Biological Actions of Dimethyl Sulfoxide* (New York Academy of Sciences, Vol. 24, eds. Stanley W. Jacob and Robert Herschler). The study was divided into two parts, both involving volunteer prisoners from the state prison hospital at Vacaville, California. One study ran for fourteen days, the other for ninety days. For each of the studies, Dr. Hull enlisted the help of area physicians, each to handle specialized examinations; and to make sure of the reliability of the ophthalmological phase of the study, he enlisted the help of a Portland, Oregon, researcher named Don Wood, who had been doing DMSO studies on dogs and understood the DMSO eye-change phenomenon.

There was nothing complicated about the study. Each of the prisoners taking part received a daily treatment of an 80 percent DMSO gel at a dosage of one gram per kilogram of body weight of the subject. This, depending on the circumstances, is from three to thirty times the normal human treatment dose. The subjects received the entire dose once a day, in multiple applications; one layer was applied. It was allowed to soak in and dry, after which other layers were applied until the daily dosage requirement was completed. Each prisoner was given a thorough physical examination prior to the DMSO treatment period and after the treatment period ended. These physical and chemical examinations were unusually thorough. They covered the blood pressure, pulse, temperature, respiration, head, ears, eyes, throat, neck, thyroid, lungs, heart, abdomen, liver, kidney, spleen, rectal system, extremities, skin and nervous system. In each instance, a specialist conducted the examination. The ophthalmological examination made use of a device known as the slit lamp, which can reveal even the slightest abnormalities in the lens of the eye. Two additional ophthalmological examinations were given to each prisoner—one two weeks after the treatment period and one four weeks after the period.

The results of both studies were the same. None of the prisoners in either study showed any serious toxic effects. And nothing turned up in the laboratory analysis of the blood that indicated a serious toxic effect. There were the predictable breath, odor and skin effects, and there were complaints from about half the prisoners about mild fatigue and headache, but no other side effects of any consequence showed up. (Significantly, although this study was done in 1967, with the close cooperation of FDA officials, some FDA officials, as recently as 1980, were issuing public statements about the possible "eye toxicity" of DMSO.)

The Vacaville study established that DMSO, when applied topically, produces no serious side effects. Furthermore, there is nothing in the animal studies, nor data from clinical reports, to indicate that DMSO is toxic in *any* modality when administered with the same care and supervision that you would expect with any therapeutic substance. "It's important to view this whole safety issue with perspective," Stanley Jacob says. "There are many pharmacological experts who will tell you that if aspirin were being introduced for the first time today, it wouldn't even get to a point at which investigators could test it on humans. The same goes for penicillin. There is no drug today that won't produce side effects if one gives a large enough dosage. What is surprising about DMSO," he observes, "is not the side effects it produces, but the fact that, even in very high dosages, it's a substance of such low toxicity."

The Eye Question

"I heard that it hurts the eyes of rabbits," basketball star Dan Issel, of the Denver Nuggets, told a *Rocky Mountain News* reporter in May, 1981. "So I don't use DMSO every week."

The possibility that DMSO is harmful to the eyes is the number one concern regarding its safety. It has been this way since 1965, when the FDA banned DMSO testing in humans on the basis of animal studies showing changes in the lenses of rabbits and other laboratory animals receiving large doses of DMSO. Almost every FDA communication regarding DMSO from that day on has talked about "toxic eye effects," and so it is no wonder that many people have come to believe that DMSO may very well pose a threat to their vision.

The facts speak otherwise.

First, the animals in the studies that promoted the FDA action in 1965 were not going "blind"; there were changes that produced near-sightedness. Second, the FDA was aware of these changes well before it issued the ban— a fact that serves to confirm Herschler and Jacob's contention that the FDA simply used the rabbit eye findings as a pretext to stop DMSO testing until the agency could gain a greater measure of control over the number of people using DMSO throughout the United States.

"This eye effect in animals is unique," says Dr. Lionel Rubin, of the school of veterinary medicine at the University of Pennsylvania, who has studied this phenomenon more thoroughly than anybody else. "No other compound has been reported to cause even a similar effect."

The effect that Rubin refers to has in the lay press often been called "cataracts," but this description is not only incorrect, it is also misleading. What happens is that when certain animals—rabbits in particular—are given high doses of DMSO, their lenses become less relucent than normal, which means a loss of some capacity to reflect light. The animals do not become blind. "What happens," says Dr. Rubin, "is that the refraction surface of the lens —the lens surface that bends during focusing—becomes more convex than normal, pushing it slightly further back in the eye than normal." The animal becomes near-sighted.

These eye changes, whatever their effect, have been shown to occur definitely in only three species: rabbits, dogs and swine. Although there is one English study that reports these changes occur in monkeys—a study the FDA refers to frequently—there are four well-controlled studies that show no such change. One of these studies was conducted by Dr. Lionel Rubin. Rubin reports that young monkeys given doses up to nine grams per kilogram of body weight per day, orally, for eighteen months, showed no changes (ten grams per kilogram would amount to 1 percent of body weight).

Dr. Rubin says he doesn't know why this ocular effect occurs, and neither does anybody else know for certain. Herschler theorizes that the effect might have to do with some disruption of microorganisms in the animals' digestive system—the result of DMSO's antimicrobial effects. But one thing is fairly certain. DMSO doesn't accumulate in the lens. Researchers know this because of experiments administering radioactively labeled DMSO. Neither is this phenomenon, whatever it is, the same thing that occurs in cataract formation.

To better relate to this DMSO effect on the lens of certain animals, one must also realize that many drugs, particularly when given at high dose levels, cause eye changes. A number of FDA-approved drugs can cause eye changes in animals at recommended dosage levels. A sizeable list of new drugs approved since 1965 by the FDA had documented eye changes in man, and far more serious toxicity problems at recommended dosages, even before approval was given. Some of these drugs are recommended treatment for disorders that one can hardly classify as life-threatening. One might then ask—why has the FDA made such a propaganda effort regarding certain eye changes seen in lower animals given DMSO, even though the effect has never been seen in man? Only the FDA can answer this question.

"I wish I had an explanation for the eye effects in animals," Stanley Jacob says, "but I don't. It's one of those things that occurs very often when you're testing drugs. An effect shows up in a species, and no one has an explanation. The important thing to remember is that in spite of what the FDA has been saying, there is not a single documented case of a person suffering a serious eye problem attributable to DMSO, and I know people who've been using it for 18 years. To the contrary," Jacob points out, "DMSO has been very effective in treating certain types of eye problems. The FDA has been trying since 1965 to find data that will support the decision it made to ban testing, and not even *their* investigators have come up with any solid evidence to show DMSO is dangerous to the human eye. You would think they'd know when to acknowledge their error."

The Genetic Effects of DMSO

As any pharmacologist will tell you, the fact that a substance doesn't have toxic effects on humans doesn't mean that it won't produce birth defects in newborns, and so a big part of drug safety testing is aimed at determining the level of a drug's teratogenicity—its toxic effects on embryos. Some press reports have suggested that DMSO causes birth defects in animals, but, here again, the preponderant facts speak otherwise. In one study, eight cell embryos were soaked in DMSO and reimplanted. All developed normally. Indeed, DMSO is by any measure one of the least embryo-toxic substances in pharmacology. It is routinely used as a solvent when scientists are studying the mutagenic effects of other drugs. DMSO's non-mutagenic effects have been confirmed by a scientist named Bruce Ames, whose test is the standard by which the FDA itself measures mutagenicity.

"There is probably no drug today," says Stanley Jacob, "that won't produce some abnormalities in newborns when you give a high enough dose, and so to say that tests show that DMSO causes birth defects is scientifically incorrect. You could probably get the same effects with many other agents. Even so, my feeling about pregnant women taking DMSO is the same as my feeling about pregnant women taking any drug not absolutely necessary to their health. They should avoid drugs if possible and never take any medication except under a doctor's supervision."

The Side Effects of DMSO

It is true that DMSO causes certain side effects, but these effects are of a "nuisance" type, and far less serious than the side effects produced by most prescription drugs.

DMSO's most troublesome side effect—that it can give you bad breath—is more social than anything else. Exactly *why* it gives you bad breath is hard to say, but there is no correlation between DMSO's breath effect and its therapeutic effectiveness. In other words, the fact that you do or don't get bad breath has nothing to do with how much relief you get from DMSO. What's more, it probably isn't so much the DMSO itself that produces the bad breath odor, but the fact that DMSO enhances whatever breath odor you normally have. For what it's worth, vegetarians, as a group, seem to have fewer complaints about the breath problem than heavy meat eaters.

There is hope on the horizon. Newer formulations of

DMSO, now being developed by Robert Herschler, have lessened the odor problem and reduced skin irritation, although it will be some time before these products are available to the general public, regardless of how the FDA rules on the original DMSO formula. In the meantime, if you take DMSO in large and regular amounts, you may have to accept the possibility of not having kissing-sweet breath. One Florida physician reports good-humoredly that he always knows, even before they tell him, when any of his patients have applied DMSO prior to a visit, and it was a standing joke among members of the UCLA football team that DMSO did wonders for your aches and pains but could just about kill your social life.

Not that the breath odor is essentially a bad thing in the minds of some physicians. Dr. Arthur Scherbel of the Cleveland Clinic, for instance, sees the odor connected with DMSO as a good control mechanism. "People will use it only when they need to use it, and won't use it when they don't need it."

Apart from the breath odor that people who take DMSO sometimes give off, the most frequently reported side effect of DMSO is a skin irritation at the site of application. There is no predictable pattern. Just as some people can take relatively large dosages of DMSO and experience neither the odor nor the taste, so do skin irritations vary from person to person. Some people can literally bathe themselves in solutions of DMSO of 70 percent or greater and experience no adverse skin reactions whatsoever. A few patients, however, break out in a rash or hives with concentrations of less than 50 percent DMSO. Dr. Marvin Paul, a Canadian physician who has long been one of DMSO's clinical investigators, suggests that people who are more prone to skin reactions are more likely than others to have skin reactions from DMSO. "I myself am very fair-skinned," he says, "and the first time I used it on my back, I did have a mild skin reaction. But the relief it gave my back was more than worth it. You have to use common sense with DMSO, but that's one of the best things about the substance. You can vary the concentration according to the needs of the patient."

Most people who apply 70 percent DMSO for the first time experience a slight stinging or burning at the application site. The sensation often changes to a slight itch that may linger for about an hour. Interestingly, however, these effects subside after a few days of continued application, which means that the skin acclimates itself to the substance.

A steady diet of DMSO to the same area of the body for several weeks will sometimes lead to a mild scaling or drying of the skin. This condition, should it happen, clears up on its own when DMSO treatment is stopped or the solution weakened. Some patients report that long-term use of DMSO actually improves dry and scaly skin.

The mechanism behind the skin reaction to DMSO is probably related to the release of histamine, a substance that cells known as mast cells release when they come into contact with an unfamiliar material. Mild histamine responses produce nothing more than a temporary redness or itching to the local area where an unfamiliar material is applied, but more serious histamine reactions can produce hives and generalized itching. "My leg itched like crazy," says a New Yorker who treated a sprained ankle by administering DMSO the way many athletes do it—to the level of skin tolerance. "I was putting the DMSO on every few hours. But once the sprain was better in three days, and I stopped the DMSO, the itching went away, and I was no worse for wear." Still, there have been a few reported cases of more systemic allergic reactions from DMSO—sneezing, itching of the eyes, and, in isolated instances, breathing difficulty. Yet, says Stanley Jacob, "I know of no substance, with the possible exception of water, "that doesn't produce an allergic reaction in at least a small proportion of the people who take it." And, he explains, "You can tell very quickly with DMSO whether you're seriously allergic to it or not, and the intelligent thing for a doctor to do when he notices any reaction that goes beyond a localized skin reaction is to suspend treatment. There's a good margin of safety."

Clinical studies on DMSO show that 50 to 75 percent of the people who take it experience one form of skin reaction or another when the strength of DMSO is 70 percent or stronger. But serious skin reactions are rare. Of the more than 10,000 patients treated with DMSO in Berlin by Heinz John and Gerhard Laudahn in the mid-1960's, only 3.5 percent experienced a local skin reaction troublesome enough that treatment had to be discontinued. (Biological Actions of DMSO, New York Academy of Science, 1967.) In every instance, according to the two German doctors, the symptoms were cleared up within ten days of treatment, with either a simple cortisone ointment or no therapy at all. Generalized skin reactions serious enough to require stopping the treatment were rarer, occurring in only 0.1 percent of the patients.

The Berlin results were corroborated in Dr. J. Harold Brown's double-blind series of tests on patients with acute musculoskeletal injuries or conditions (see chapter III). Dr. Brown found that while 15 percent of his patients had "marked" skin reactions to DMSO, none of the reactions was serious enough to require suspending the treatment.

Is DMSO Safe?

Bearing in mind what both Jacob and Herschler have been saying all along—that no drug is without side effects —we can draw the following general conclusions with respect to the safety of DMSO:

Relative to most drugs, including aspirin, DMSO has a low level of toxicity. The FDA acknowledges this. So does the National Academy of Sciences.

The side effects that DMSO produces are more irritating than they are serious. The two main side effects are breath odor and mild skin reactions at the point of application.

The animal studies that led the FDA to ban testing of DMSO on humans concern changes in the lenses of certain animals. But this phenomenon has not yet been discovered in humans, even though there are a great many people who have been using DMSO regularly for nearly twenty years.

"My position on the safety of DMSO is simply this," says Jacob. "I think it's one of the safest compounds ever developed. Even so, because it's a drug and because every drug has some side effects, people should always check with a doctor before using it, and should always use it under a doctor's supervision."

CHAPTER X

The Politics of
DMSO

If everything had gone according to the way Robert Herschler and Stanley Jacob figured it would go when they made their initial discoveries about DMSO, here, in rough outline, is what would have taken place over the past two decades.

First of all, as is customary with new scientific discoveries, Herschler and Jacob would have published their early findings in one of the important scientific journals, the editors of which would have recognized immediately that Herschler and Jacob had made a medical discovery of historic importance. These papers would have excited other scientists and physicians to conduct studies on their own —studies that would have confirmed Herschler and Jacob's findings. Still other scientists would have launched their own DMSO studies, making new discoveries and publishing these findings in further papers. There would have been a flurry of DMSO symposia—gatherings at which scientists and physicians would have read papers and exchanged ideas about DMSO and its therapeutic potential.

While the scientific community was exploring the medical potential of DMSO, the drug industry would have been taking advantage of its commercial potential. The drug companies, of course, would have taken DMSO through the normal testing procedures, the better to demonstrate to the FDA that it was safe and effective, and the approval process, in all likelihood, would have taken as long as two to three years. But, in due time, approval would have come, and DMSO probably would have made its initial appearance on the drug market as a prescriptive gel, for use in the treatment of acute injuries such as sprains, burns and contusions. New DMSO products would have quickly followed: DMSO in various solutions for various types of conditions in various types of administrations: antibiotic mixtures made up partly of DMSO; anti-inflammatory substances with DMSO; dermatological medications containing DMSO. Conceivably, too, cancer chemotherapy would today reflect the influence of DMSO, through the mixing of DMSO with anti-cancer drugs so as to cut down on the amount of these drugs that had to be used—so cutting down on their side effects—without sacrificing their potency.

As DMSO became more widely used and more widely understood, more and more researchers in different specialties in medicine would have begun DMSO-related studies. Moreover, it is not inconceivable that by the mid-1970's, for example, the safety and effectiveness of DMSO for general medical purposes would have been so well established that the FDA would have lifted its prescription-only status for certain forms of DMSO, so that you could buy it over-the-counter.

All of this would mean that today, if you wanted to use DMSO for any number of conditions—an ankle sprain, arthritic pain, a bad burn, sinusitis or whatever—you wouldn't have to go to a veterinarian for it, or have to buy it as a solvent for twenty times what it costs to produce. You could simply walk into your local drugstore and, for the price of a bottle of aspirin or a tube of Ben-Gay, buy enough DMSO to last you a month or two. DMSO would be as ubiquitous in its medical uses, in other words, as aspirin. It would indeed be the "aspirin of the twenty-first century."

So much for what *might* have happened to DMSO during the two decades that followed Robert Herschler's initial discoveries. What *has* happened is a sequence of depressing and often incredible events that even in retrospect is difficult for the people most closely involved with DMSO to understand. As Herschler now puts it, "If there is such a thing as a Murphy's law of new drug development, DMSO proves it. Everything that could go wrong did go wrong."

The trouble began as soon as Herschler and Jacob tried to publish their initial findings. In their first paper, they listed what they had found to be the seven primary pharmacological actions of DMSO: the fact that it could (1) penetrate membranes; (2) reduce pain; (3) reduce inflammation; (4) inhibit bacterial growth; (5) promote diuresis; (6) act as a tranquilizer; and (7) potentiate other compounds. But none of the scientific journals to which they submitted the paper shared Herschler's and Jacob's belief that DMSO was a medical discovery of major importance. What's more, whenever Jacob would talk to his colleagues about DMSO, he ran into much the same kind of resistance. Most people found it ludicrous that a common industrial solvent could do everything that Herschler and Jacob were saying it could do. Herschler's superiors at Crown Zellerbach thought he was wasting his time and refused to provide any support to further his research. Some of Jacob's colleagues at the University of Oregon thought he'd gone off the deep end. "It was a very frustrating experience," Herschler says. "Stanley and I knew what we were seeing with our own eyes, and we were both convinced that we had found something truly unique, truly remarkable. We wanted to share our excitement with other scientists and other physicians, and people kept slamming the door in our face."

Part of the explanation for what Herschler and Jacob were running into is that science and medicine are not as receptive to innovation as you might think, based on the rate of scientific development in this century. As the history of medicine shows, nearly every major medical advance—the idea of sterilizing instruments before surgery, to cite just one example—has been initially dismissed and resisted by the medical establishment. What's more, important medical journals are reluctant to publish reports of any clinical findings with obvious and immediate application to widespread diseases and conditions for which there is no truly effective treatment, for the editors know that the lay press is forever looking for stories of medical "breakthroughs." Indeed, the more obvious the therapeutic benefit of a discovery, the harder it is to get a scientific journal to publish the study, unless you can show irrefutable and compelling evidence to back up your claims. Herschler and Jacob had done a number of studies, but lacked the resources to conduct the kind of long-term clinical studies and animal studies that would have been necessary to satisfy the editors of certain publications. Nonetheless, patients Jacob was treating were experiencing dramatic relief, and, in many cases, in conditions for which there wasn't any truly effective and safe medication. "From the beginning," says Jacob, "the incredible thing about DMSO is that you didn't have to do a bunch of tests on animals to see if it worked or not. You could *demonstrate* it. If you put DMSO on a black eye, you could *see* a difference within an hour. I fully accept the concept that drugs have to be tested to make sure they're safe, but the idea that we had to run tests in animals to show that DMSO could do things we could dramatically see in human patients didn't strike me as being very efficient."

Eventually, a paper on DMSO made its way into the scientific literature, in a journal called *Current Therapeutic Research*. The paper was submitted in 1963 but not published until early 1964. In the meantime, the lay press had gotten wind of the DMSO story. On December 10, 1963, two Portland newspapers ran a story of a meeting that had taken place between officials of Crown Zellerbach and officials of the Board of Higher Education of Oregon. The purpose of the meeting was to formalize a patent agreement whereby Herschler's employer, Crown Zellerbach, and Jacob's employer, the Board of Higher Education, would share any patent-derived royalties that might accrue from the discovery that DMSO had drug usefulness. But in addition to reporting on the meeting, both articles described DMSO and listed its basic medical properties. DMSO, so to speak, was out of the bag.

To this day, Robert Herschler and Stanley Jacob insist they did nothing to instigate these newspaper articles, and there is no reason to believe otherwise. To the contrary, both men would have much preferred that the lay press not publish anything about DMSO until *after* their findings had been published in a scientific journal. And for a good reason: there is an unwritten rule in the scientific and medical communities that reports of new discoveries should be kept out of the public eye until the discoveries have been validated by qualified scientists and physicians.

That neither Herschler nor Jacob had any hand in orchestrating the first article in the lay press was of little consequence to many of their scientific and medical colleagues. They had "broken the rules." They were immediately accused in some circles of being opportunists, more interested in making money and advancing their own interests than they were in science. To this day, in fact, there are doctors and scientists who are ill-disposed to DMSO for no other reason than that the first reports of its medical properties appeared not in a scientific journal but in a local Portland, Oregon, newspaper.

To make matters even worse, as far as Jacob and Herschler were concerned, *The New York Times* picked up on the Portland story and a week later ran an account of its own, with the headline "Multi-Purpose Drug Reported on the Coast." The article quoted a physician at the medical school—not Dr. Jacob—as saying that he'd used DMSO on a dozen patients and considered it "the most exciting thing he'd seen in medicine." Among its other effects, the *New York Times* report sent Crown Zellerbach stock from $4.50 a share up to $60.25, although the rush to buy the stock cooled when company executives made a public statement to the effect that commercialization of DMSO for medical purposes would have little effect on its overall sales, volume and profits.

Yet according to Robert Herschler, who was there at the time, some executives—while Crown Zellerbach was issuing public statements about how little DMSO would mean to their balance sheet—were actively drumming up publicity for DMSO among the publishers of several leading magazines. "Crown Zellerbach had almost no sensitivity about the problems that arise when the lay press gets hold of a big medical story too soon," says Herschler. "They were in the paper business, not the drug business. They figured DMSO was just like any other product—that publicity would be good for it."

In any case, articles on DMSO began appearing in several major magazines, among them *Time, Newsweek, Life,* the *Saturday Evening Post* and *Pageant*—even though DMSO had not been adequately tested and wasn't even available in medicinal form. "We never solicited any of these articles," laments Jacobs. "Most of the time, nobody at the University was even consulted. Any time a reporter asked me a question about DMSO, I went out of my way to underplay the drug. Bob and I both saw what was happening and we were both concerned. We didn't *want* the publicity."

If the growing public interest in DMSO was spooky to Herschler and Jacob, it had the effect of a supercharged cattle prod on the drug industry. True, none of the drug companies owned the patent on the medical uses of DMSO, but a drug company can still earn a lot of money on a drug with a wide enough market, whether it holds the patent or not. The company simply makes a licensing arrangement, whereby it agrees to give a certain percentage of sales to the patent holder. "All the major drug companies saw enormous potential in DMSO," says Herschler. "They were excited about the drug. They saw it as the sort of substance that every man, woman and child might have use for. They saw it, really, as another aspirin."

Backing up Herschler's view is the fact that no fewer than thirty different drug companies dispatched representatives to Portland in early 1964 to seek licenses from Crown Zellerbach. Here again, it appears that Crown Zellerbach's inexperience served DMSO a crippling disservice. "If Crown had handled the thing intelligently," says Herschler, "they would have picked one or two companies at the most—which is what I was urging them to do. In that way they could have controlled the testing phase of the approval process and wouldn't have run into problems with the FDA." But Crown Zellerbach officials ignored Herschler's advice and awarded licenses to six of the world's largest companies: Merck, Sharpe and Dohme, E. R. Squibb & Sons, American Home Products, Syntex, Geigy and Schering. Shortly thereafter, an additional license was given to Schering A.G. in Europe.

What followed the awarding of these multiple licenses is described by Robert Herschler as a "fiasco." Several of the companies, determined to be the first to bring out a DMSO product, committed millions of dollars and immediately began recruiting physician-investigators to set up and conduct the safety and effectiveness studies. None of the companies was doing anything wrong, but there was an atmosphere of urgency about the whole affair that was worrisome to a lot of people.

"It was a very unhealthy situation," recalls Herschler. "The testing got out of control because of the competition. The worst of it was that it scared the FDA. They'd never had to deal with this kind of situation before, with so many drug companies involved in studies on the same drug, and with all the public pressure that was building."

It didn't help matters, either, that less than two years earlier, as a result of the thalidomide disaster, Congress had passed a law that gave the FDA a good deal of latitude in establishing safety- and effectiveness-testing procedures.

Among other things, the law led the FDA to establish rigid—many would argue impossible—new approval standards. Prior to 1962, the FDA was concerned mainly with the safety of drugs, but the FDA's actions with respect to the 1962 Kefauver-Harris Amendment to the Food, Drug and Cosmetic Act put a herculean burden on the drug companies to produce "substantial" evidence that a drug was effective as well. It also gave to the FDA far more power than it had earlier had to control the testing procedures—it could, for all intents, now set up its own measures of effectiveness independent of the scientific and medical community. "The FDA took a law that was set up to protect the public and used it as a pretext to control the way medicine is practiced in the United States," maintains Robert Herschler.

With thalidomide still fresh in the public eye, most Americans believed that the new FDA regulations were a good and necessary thing. Better, after all, to be safe than

sorry. But what most Americans didn't know at the time
—and still don't know—is that the drug approval process
in the United States was about to become a bureaucratic
Frankenstein—so much so that the number of new medications available to Americans would drop from an average of forty-three a year in the ten years prior to 1962 to
less than thirteen a year from 1972 to the present. At the
same time, the cost of taking a new drug through the mul-
ti-phase FDA testing merry-go-round was to soar into the
tens of millions of dollars (the ultimate price borne by the
consumer who pays for prescription drugs), while the
amount of paperwork a drug company would have to
submit when seeking approval would become so volumi-
nous that material meant to be reviewed must now often
be hand-trucked into the office of the medical reviewer.
And a company submitting an NDA (a new drug application) that could at one time have been expected to get
FDA approval within six months was to eventually have
to wait an average of two to three years.

"What has happened with the FDA since 1962," says
Stanley Jacob, "is similar to what happens in medicine a
lot of time. The 'cure' has been worse than the disease. We
need a system in this country for determining the safety
and effectiveness of drugs. What we don't need is a government agency whose actions are penalizing the public
by discouraging the drug companies from developing new
medications in this country."

In one way or another, every new drug that has been introduced since 1962 has been victimized to some extent
by the new FDA regulations, but probably no drug has
been victimized more than DMSO. "Bob and I could sense
from the start," says Jacob, "that the FDA simply didn't
know how to handle DMSO. I can remember very clearly
a meeting in March at which one of the FDA officials—
Dr. Frances Kelsey—told us they were very concerned
over the possibility that they'd be overwhelmed with

DMSO-related New Drug Applications. They didn't know how they were going to control the testing process. And that's been the issue from the beginning—not whether DMSO is safe or not, or whether it works or not, but whether the FDA is calling all the shots."

Still, as apprehensive as both Jacob and Herschler may have been during the early stages of the FDA-required studies, they had reason for being optimistic. Preliminary reports from Merck, Sharpe and Dohme investigators were verifying everything that Herschler and Jacob had been saying all along about DMSO. DMSO did indeed, a Merck, Sharpe and Dohme report confirmed, relieve pain and inflammation and did indeed inhibit the growth of bacteria. DMSO also penetrated membranes and showed clinical effectiveness in the treatment of sprains, sinusitis, gout and a number of other conditions, said the Merck report. What's more, Merck investigators listed as side effects of DMSO nothing that Jacob and Herschler hadn't themselves known about: the funny taste, bad breath, some redness and itching at the point of application.

Only one finding in the Merck report came as a surprise. Some investigators working with animals found that curious changes occurred in the lenses of the eyes of rabbits and dogs given high doses of DMSO. Eye effects in animals are hardly unusual when you conduct the kind of high-dosage toxicity tests that investigators conduct to determine the safety of a drug. In fact, most of the investigators working on DMSO at Merck had observed far more serious eye changes when testing drugs that were currently on the market, and so no one was pushing the panic button—particularly since none of the humans involved in the clinical testing of DMSO were complaining of eye problems or showing any eye effects. "We all knew about the eye findings," Jacob says. "The Merck, Sharpe and Dohme investigators felt that the best way to handle the situation was to advise people using DMSO on a long-term basis to have periodic eye examinations. The FDA had the findings as early as spring, 1965, as part of Merck, Sharpe and Dohme's NDA. It was all very routine. As far as everybody was concerned, the studies couldn't have been going any better."

Not quite. For trouble during this period was brewing on other fronts. One problem was that all the publicity about DMSO (the result of the many articles appearing in national magazines) was generating an avalanche of public pressure to make DMSO available. In February, 1965, a Merck, Sharpe and Dohme executive told Stanley Jacob that the company was getting more requests from people wanting the drug than they'd had for any other drug they'd ever developed. At the same time many people were using DMSO who, by FDA rules, weren't supposed to be using it until it received the agency's seal of approval. Most were getting it from chemical supply houses that were selling DMSO as a solvent. Doctors who weren't official investigators were giving it to patients. "It was a very hard thing to control," says Jacob. "People would get DMSO, use it on themselves, tell other people about it. The important thing to remember, though, is that people were being helped by it. If DMSO was dangerous, we would have known very quickly."

The FDA didn't see things quite the same way. By the spring of 1965, as many as 100,000 Americans were using a substance that the FDA had yet to certify as safe and effective. Big-name athletes were using it. So were movie stars. And there was nothing the FDA could say or do to keep people from getting DMSO on their own. "We knew the FDA was getting edgy," Jacob says, "but we also felt the data we were getting from the various drug company investigators were solid enough that DMSO was safe and effective. What we didn't know was the FDA at this time was more concerned with its regulations than it was with finding out the human benefits of the drug."

In early September, 1965, two months after Jacob took part in the first international symposium on DMSO, DMSO became a prescription drug in Germany. At around the same time, Dr. J. Harold Brown presented a report of a double blind-type study of DMSO before the Washington State Medical Society, in which he told his fellow physicians that as far as he was concerned DMSO was so effective a treatment medium for soft-tissue injuries that he had abandoned what he termed "antedated treatment." "I have discontinued all analgesics, muscle relaxants, tranquilizers, corticosteroids and physical therapy," Dr. Brown told the astonished group. "My results with DMSO were dramatic and striking."

Dr. Brown's talk, coming on the heels of the German decision to okay DMSO as a prescription drug, was, as Herschler and Jacob remember it, the "high point" with regard to their hopes for DMSO. But the euphoria didn't last long. On September 9, 1965, an article in the *Wall Street Journal* reported that a forty-four-year-old woman in Ireland had died while taking DMSO. As it happens, the woman was on a number of medications at the time she was taking DMSO, any one of which could have produced an allergic reaction, and since no autopsy was performed, there was no reason for suspecting DMSO to be the cause of the woman's death. Indeed, it was never established that the woman's death was drug related. In any case, the FDA immediately dispatched telegrams to an estimated 1,000 investigators who were treating humans with DMSO—with warnings about its possible "lethal effects."

The next thing the FDA did was take action against Crown Zellerbach. Crown Zellerbach was conducting clinical tests, but not with the idea of developing a specific drug product. It was doing the testing basically as an added measure of insurance to solidify its patent rights. As Robert Herschler subsequently discovered, the company didn't need to conduct clinical studies on humans to satisfy patent requirements: animal studies would have served a better purpose. "I was against the idea of Crown Zellerbach getting involved in clinical testing," says Herschler. "It was a major business blunder. They had no idea of how to control the studies and they left themselves wide open to FDA attack. I urged my superiors on many occasions in 1965 to stop the testing, that the tests weren't necessary and that the company didn't know what it was doing."

As things happened, the FDA itself put Crown Zellerbach out of the testing business, accusing the company of "violating FDA regulations." This was the first of a series of official actions that the FDA would take against DMSO, whose sum effect would be to discredit the drug in the eyes of the public and the scientific community.

But the worst was yet to come. On November 11, 1965, representatives from each of the drug companies that had investigators doing studies on DMSO were summoned to Washington for a meeting whose stated purpose, according to the FDA, was to discuss "eye changes" in laboratory animals. By bureaucratic standards, it was a short meeting and there was no "discussion." Once the representatives had gathered in an FDA conference room, Dr. Joseph F. Sadusk, Jr., then the medical director of the FDA, walked in with about two dozen other FDA administrators and read to the assembled group a telegram. The telegram advised any physician who was testing DMSO on humans to suspend the testing. The drug companies were told by the FDA to send each of their investigators a copy. The telegrams went out that day, in addition to which the FDA sent the same telegram to the World Health Organization and American embassies throughout the world.

News of the FDA decision to halt testing of DMSO on humans shook both Herschler and Jacob, but they took solace in their belief that the agency had simply taken a temporary action whose purpose was to get the testing procedures under control. "I figured the thing would cool down in a few months," Herschler says, "so I didn't let myself get too disappointed."

"I felt the same way," Jacob says. "I believed the eye question wasn't serious," he adds, "and I knew the FDA knew this. I figured that after a short period, we'd be on track again. We were a little naive, to say the least."

Naive is hardly the word for it. For not only did the FDA not lift the ban within a few months, so that the testing process could go on, it chose to relax the ban in limited stages. In 1966, they granted to investigators who were so inclined the right to conduct limited studies on conditions for which there was no known cure. Two years later, following an extensive toxicity study among inmates at a California prison, the FDA said it was all right to test for other conditions, but insisted on a certain protocol—frequent eye examinations during the testing period—that served to complicate an already complicated treatment procedure. Indeed, it wasn't until 1980 that the FDA removed all the restraints it had put on the testing of DMSO in humans, thus restoring DMSO to the status of any experimental drug.

The FDA's public position throughout this period has been to depict itself as a kind of public watch dog, serving an important function, doing its job well, refusing to bend to "pressures" that would jeopardize the public interest. "People should be protected from unsafe and ineffective drugs," former FDA Commissioner Jere Goyan said during one Senate subcommittee hearing on DMSO; "the FDA has a statutory and public health obligation to approve only those drugs that have been shown by scientific evidence to be safe and effective. The law containing these principles of safety and effectiveness is a good law," he stated, adding that "the Congress and the public should be proud of its existence and should reject any attempts to weaken or undermine it."

As far as the FDA is concerned, the primary reason that DMSO is not an approved drug for any condition apart from interstitial cystitis (this approval, for a 50 percent DMSO solution, came in 1978), is that its safety and effectiveness have yet to be shown through "well-controlled" studies. True, the FDA concedes, there are thousands of personal testimonies suggesting that DMSO is effective, and there have been hundreds of studies on it conducted throughout the world, but the vast majority of these studies, the FDA maintains, do not meet FDA "control" criteria.

"The fundamental problem from our point of view," Dr. Richard J. Crout, former director of the Bureau of Drugs of the FDA, told a House subcommittee in March, 1980, "is the quality of the scientific information available to support the various claims that are made for DMSO." Dr. Crout then went on to say that the FDA is as anxious as anybody to make available to the American people any substance that could represent a major medical advance, but that most of the evidence that points up DMSO's effectiveness is of dubious scientific value. "The FDA," he said, "is willing, indeed anxious, to approve DMSO for any uses whenever controlled trials meeting the statutory standard are available. We have worked in the past, and stand ready to work in the future, with any party in developing protocols for such trials and in expediting their review."

Apart from their insistence that DMSO has yet to "prove" itself by acceptable scientific standards, FDA officials have been arguing for years that supporters of DMSO have been doing their best to circumvent the law by which the FDA draws its power. Thus, although

DMSO has been widely promoted for arthritis, the FDA claims that currently no drug company has even seen fit to submit to the FDA and IND for the treatment of arthritis with DMSO. More serious, in the minds of some FDA officials, is that some of the investigators working with DMSO have not only ignored FDA regulations in the testing process, but have gone so far as to conceal findings that might cast an unfavorable light on DMSO's safety and effectiveness.

It's a strong argument and one that would appear, on the surface at least, to have a good deal of merit. But the FDA's public position fails to acknowledge a number of crucial aspects of the DMSO situation that give the DMSO controversy a much different perspective than the FDA would like the public to have.

In the first place, the FDA's 1965 decision to ban further human testing of DMSO ostensibly because of its eye effects in lower animals was an all but mortal wound to the development of DMSO as a drug. The only way a drug can get FDA approval in the United States for *any* usage is on the basis of studies funded and carried out by drug companies. But since 1965 none of the major drug companies, not even any of the companies involved in the initial studies, has been willing to make a major financial commitment to DMSO, given the cost of drug development in general and the fact that the FDA has hardly shown itself to be enthusiastic about DMSO. "The drug companies are scared to death of the FDA," says a leading executive for a major pharmaceutical firm on the East Coast. "If an FDA official wants to," says the executive, "he can slow up the approval procedure by months and even years, and increase the developmental cost of a drug by millions of dollars. And there's almost nothing you can do about it." Robert Herschler adds: "If *you* were the president of a drug company, and you had to commit as much as $70 million to bring to the market a substance that's already been maliciously scored before the approval process began, what would *you* do?"

The FDA ban also effectively scared away private researchers, most of whom depend on government funding for their research. Scientists who know their way around the government machinery are smart enough to know that you're better off working in areas in which there is no danger of political fallout.

A third problem FDA officials do not mention when they discuss DMSO in public is that the kind of controls they talk about in scientific studies are next to impossible to apply to a substance as easily detectable as DMSO. Ideally, when the FDA talks about "well-controlled" studies, it is talking about so-called "double-blind studies," in which neither the scientists administering a substance nor the patients taking it know whether it is actually the substance being tested, another medication, or a placebo. The purpose of these "blind" controls is to make sure that "nonscientific" factors don't color the final results. The patients cannot "imagine" that they are getting better, since they do not know whether or not they are truly receiving a drug, or merely a placebo. The investigators cannot affect the results through any power of suggestion. The results become known only when scientists who hold the "key" —or code—to which substance was given to which patient reveal this. And they do not do this until all of the medical results of the study have been gathered.

"Because of the taste you get from DMSO and the smell it has, it's very difficult to set up classic double-blind protocols with the drug," explains Stanley Jacob. "What the FDA doesn't say, though, is that most of the prescription drugs that have been on the market for years and have proven themselves to be safe and effective didn't have to meet the double-blind protocol standards. There are other ways you can prove the effectiveness of a drug without getting mired down in the technicalities of how 'controlled' the studies have been. The studies that have been done on DMSO—and there have been thousands of them —have been carried out by careful scientists and at some of the most prestigious scientific and medical centers in the world," he explains. "We're not talking about a 'laetrile' here. We're talking about one of the most exhaustively studied drugs in the history of medicine."

But forgetting for the moment the question of controls and scientific protocols, it is Herschler and Jacob's conviction that most of the FDA actions involving DMSO since 1965 have been designed to justify the decision made that year to halt the testing on humans, and not to arrive at any definitive answers with respect to the drug's safety and effectiveness. "I was told by somebody in the FDA who was there at the time," Jacob testified before government officials in 1980, "that very shortly after they issued the ban in 1965, FDA investigators from all over the country were called to Washington and were told, in effect, to go out and 'get something' on DMSO, to 'find us some pigeons.' The FDA launched at that time what was—and what still is—the largest investigation of its kind in history. It was so big they had to bring the FBI in. So here you have a government agency whose job is to evaluate test data, going out and spending millions of dollars of tax money in order to *find* something negative about a drug —simply to back up a decision that they shouldn't have made in the first place. Here is a medical Watergate."

Stanley Jacob, of course, hardly qualifies as an unbiased observer, but a careful look at much of what has happened with DMSO since 1965 lends a disturbing amount of credence to his views. For one thing, the FDA in the early 1960's approved the anti-inflammatory drug indomethacin on the basis of studies that had protocols similar to those studies that have been submitted on DMSO. "If you compare the studies submitted on behalf of DMSO—a drug that didn't get FDA approval in 1965–," Jacob says, "with the studies submitted on behalf of Indocin around the same time, you will see very clearly that from the start the FDA has had a double standard: one for other drugs, and one for DMSO."

It must also be said that—even granting the FDA's suspicions that its regulations had been flouted by DMSO investigators—the agency has taken an unusually aggressive tack in its treatment of many DMSO investigators. Under normal circumstances, for instance, FDA investigators almost never pay personal visits to the offices of physicians who are conducting studies on drugs for which FDA approval is being sought; the agency simply doesn't have the manpower. Yet several DMSO investigators have been subjected to unannounced "inspections," not once but several times. One of the doctors involved in the studies that led to the approval of DMSO for interstitial cystitis has been "blacklisted" by the FDA—a designation which means that the FDA will not allow drug companies to use that doctor as an investigator in clinical studies. Stanley Jacob has himself been threatened with the same action, although no official blacklisting has taken place. On the other hand, Jacob discovered during two FDA "inspections" that investigators were making copies of his *private* correspondence and his files. "I still have trouble believing it," he says. "Where in our Constitution does it say that a government agency has the right to come into a doctor's office, demand copies of patient files and then start to surreptitiously copy personal correspondence."

Why would the FDA take such action? In Robert Herschler's view, the agency is simply running scared and has been using whatever tactics it can use to intimidate anybody whose involvement with DMSO might expose the agency's inept handling of DMSO from the beginning. "They jumped the gun in 1965," Herschler says. "Whatever their motives were, they quickly realized that the 'eye

toxicity' they were talking about wouldn't hold up, but instead of admitting the error, they've done everything they
can do to discredit DMSO in other ways, even to the point
of trying to ruin the reputations of people who believe in
the drug."

Herschler theorizes, too, that whether the FDA is willing to admit it or not, it is afraid of DMSO. "The public,"
he says, "knows how inexpensive DMSO is to produce.
But when you figure the amount of money it now costs a
company to steer a drug through the FDA approval process, it's going to cost the consumer a lot of money. People
are going to start to wonder about the system, and the
FDA is going to have to explain why a drug company has
to invest so much money to get approval. They stand a
chance of losing a lot of their power, and they're afraid of
it."

Whether Herschler is correct or not in his reading of the
FDA's motives, the fact remains that there are some very
basic issues involved here. Does the FDA, or any federal
agency for that matter, have the right to dictate to a doctor what that doctor can or can't prescribe to a patient, as-
suming a patient wants a particular medication? Does the
government have the right to prevent an individual from
using a substance that brings that person relief unavailable anywhere else? "The real question here," says Stanley
Jacob, "isn't whether or not there should be a mechanism
by which you can determine the safety and effectiveness
of drugs before they're available for general use. The
question is whether the mechanism we now have—the
FDA—is working to the benefit of the public."

Jacob contends that, apart from everything else, the
FDA is hidebound by its own structure and the job it has
to do. "As long as they're dealing with a single pill that
has a single effect," he says, "the machinery works. But
when you give them a substance like DMSO that has a lot
of different effects, they just don't know what to do with

it. For years, they've been trying to make DMSO conform to *their* regulations, but it's like trying to stick a square peg into a round hole—it doesn't go."

Another complaint from Jacob is that even in those instances in which he and other investigators have worked closely with FDA officials to set up studies that would meet FDA criteria for "controlled" evidence, the FDA has not been cooperative. He points out, for example, that in 1974 he and Dr. Arthur Scherbel of the Cleveland Clinic —one of the world's most respected rheumatologists and a leading authority on the disease known as scleroderma— went to the FDA in order to set up a protocol that could eventually bring about approval for DMSO in scleroderma. "We followed the protocol agreed upon," he says. "We submitted data in 1979, and it was turned down. It was turned down even though we showed that DMSO can heal the ulcers that might otherwise force a scleroderma patient to undergo amputation. Why was it turned down? Because the FDA review committee said they didn't like the protocol," explains Jacob. "When I argued that it was the FDA, along with the National Academy of Sciences, that helped us set up the protocol, we were told that all that was three or four years ago and it had nothing to do with today."

As Jacob sees it, the real reason the FDA turned down the scleroderma NDA in 1979 had nothing to do with the protocol; rather, it had to do with the FDA's realization that once a 70 percent DMSO solution were approved for DMSO, this would enable doctors to start prescribing DMSO for arthritis or, for that matter, any other condition. "There are FDA officials," Jacob says, "who are determined that nobody is going to use DMSO *legally* for arthritis unless a drug company goes through all the normal procedures. So what they're doing is playing a game—a dangerous game with people's lives. Anybody willing to look objectively at all the data that we've collected on

DMSO can't help but conclude that DMSO is not only a safe but a very effective and important medical substance."

It is difficult to predict what, exactly, will happen to DMSO over the next few years. The drug is already a prescriptive drug in a number of different forms in many countries throughout the world, among them Germany, Switzerland, Spain and the Soviet Union. And although, as of June, 1981, DMSO was a legally approved drug in the United States for only one condition, interstitial cystitis, and in only one strength—50 percent—there has been a great deal of activity on state legislative fronts. In a growing number of states, statutes already give doctors the right to prescribe DMSO in any strength and for any condition, provided that the DMSO is manufactured within state boundaries. Some states are even considering legislation that would legalize DMSO not only as a prescriptive drug but as an over-the-counter medication. The logic behind this thinking is that as long as people are buying DMSO illegally, paying black-market prices and not being able to know for certain how pure the substance is, why not offer it to them in an inexpensive and guaranteed pure form.

In the meantime, the DMSO black market continues to mushroom. At last look, DMSO at 100 percent strength was being sold at anywhere from fifteen to thirty dollars a pint—a good thirty times the cost of producing it. It is being peddled in health food stores, pharmacies, hardware stores and, in some cases, in massage parlors.

To complicate a complex situation even more, there are several investigations currently involving the FDA, the Justice Department and a number of principals involved in the development of DMSO, among them Robert Herschler and Stanley Jacob. The FDA is contending that Stanley Jacob, among others, withheld from the FDA a physician's report that spoke of eye problems with some of the patients involved in a scleroderma study. "The charge," Jacob says, "is simply not true. First of all, we showed the letter to an FDA official and were told simply to reduce the dosage on these patients and to formally submit the letter to the FDA, which we did. The important thing, though, is that we had every one of those patients examined by eye specialists and were able to show without any question that the eye problems they were having were a symptom of the disease and had nothing to do with DMSO." Jacob says that he is more than willing to testify under oath that at no time has he ever tried to conceal any evidence that might suggest that DMSO is unsafe. "What would it gain me?" he says. "If DMSO was proved to be dangerous to humans, I would be the first person to make known these dangers. I'm a physician. I'm trained to heal people—not to make them sick."

Which, of course, introduces again the question of why the FDA would make allegations and institute a Justice Department action—a question that Senator Edward Kennedy posed to Stanley Jacob at the July, 1980, Senate subcommittee hearing. "Why the agency would make allegations and representations that factual misstatements and alterations had been made in order to deny the American people the kind of relief that we heard of from the first panel of witnesses today is something I am not able to understand or comprehend," said the senator. "But," he asked Jacob, "you believe that they have."

"Yes, sir, I do," responded Jacob.

"You believe that *very* strongly?" asked Kennedy.

"Yes, sir," answered Stanley Jacob.

CHAPTER XI

===============

The Most Frequently Asked Questions about DMSO

For reasons this book has tried to make clear, there is considerable confusion in the public mind about DMSO: what it does, how it works, and why it hasn't yet been approved for wider uses. Here is a list of the most frequently asked questions about DMSO, and their answers.

What is DMSO?

DMSO is an abbreviation for dimethyl sulfoxide, a chemical compound that has been used since the mid-1950's as a commercial solvent in many industries, but has come into increasingly wide use since the early 1960's as a therapeutic agent in the treatment of many medical conditions and diseases.

What is the difference between "commercial grade"
DMSO and "pharmaceutical grade" DMSO?

The therapeutic effects are the same, providing there is
no difference in solution strength. The chief difference is
that pharmaceutical grade DMSO has undergone an extra
step in processing that rids it of the traces of other chemicals that sometimes accumulate during the normal course
of processing.

Are the impurities in commercial grade DMSO
dangerous?

Generally speaking, no. Ordinary water, in fact, con-
tains many of the same types of impurities. However,
it is possible that the containers used to store "commercial
grade" DMSO may themselves contain materials which,
taken into the body, could cause adverse reactions. To be
absolutely certain of the purity of the DMSO, use only
DMSO that has been certified as prescriptive for human
or veterinarian use.

How can you be sure the DMSO you're using is
chemically pure?

Outside of chemical analysis, it's impossible for the average person to ascertain the concentration of DMSO.
However, there are ways of getting a general idea of the
solution strength. Usually, the more water in the solution,
the more resistant to freezing the solution will be. One
way to tell whether DMSO is 99 percent strength or
greater is to place it, in its container, in the refrigerator.
It will freeze quickly if it is that strength. It takes other,
more sophisticated tests to determine the exact constitution of a DMSO-water solution below 99 percent range.

Will DMSO be spoiled if it freezes?

No. DMSO can be repeatedly frozen and thawed without affecting its purity or its therapeutic properties.

What is the difference between the various solutions of DMSO?

The higher the percentage factor, the greater is the concentration of DMSO, as opposed to water, in a solution. Higher concentration strength DMSO (70 to 90 percent) is more effective when it is applied directly to the skin, but is also likely to cause mild skin irritations. Lower concentration strengths produce very mild skin reactions, but do not have the osmotic potential to penetrate the skin rapidly. The 90 percent DMSO may be more effective in relieving some types of pain than 70 percent, but the potential for skin irritation is greater.

What is the mechanism by which DMSO works?

Because it has so many different pharmacological properties, it is impossible to state in one sentence the mechanisms by which DMSO produces its effects in the body. For instance, although its pain-relieving benefits may be tied to its ability to inhibit the firing of C-fibers, no one has pinpointed the specific analgesic mechanism of the substance. Again, DMSO's ability to permeate biological membranes may be linked to the similarities it has with water. But, once more, no definitive mechanism has been recognized. The most intelligent explanation of DMSO's overall therapeutic effect is that it promotes healing through a homeostatic mechanism, stimulating a variety of normal body processes that help to offset the attack waged by diseases.

What is the best way to use DMSO?

The "best" way to use DMSO depends upon what your problem is and how you yourself react to DMSO: your doctor is probably the best judge. Veteran DMSO users apply it topically with their fingers, using about a tablespoon for an average application for pain. There is no need to rub DMSO in; it should simply be applied to a wide area around the part of your body that's in pain. Athletes with sprained ankles usually apply DMSO over the entire foot and lower leg up to the knee. For lower-back pain, some people apply DMSO from their shoulders to their mid-thighs. If your doctor is familiar with DMSO, he'll adjust the treatment to one that works most effectively for you.

What is the best way to apply DMSO topically?

Experienced DMSO users employ their own hands to apply DMSO. Apply it liberally over a very wide area around the problem site. The difficulty with using DMSO on a cotton ball or gauze pad is that the material absorbs some of the DMSO. Consult your doctor.

What do you do with the DMSO you get on your hands once you apply it?

Rinsing your hands with water will remove any recently applied DMSO.

Why are many physicians reluctant to prescribe or recommend DMSO to their patients?

While there are physicians who frankly doubt the effectiveness and question the safety of DMSO, the majority of physicians are simply reluctant to recommend or prescribe any substance not specifically approved for the treatment of a particular disease. Some doctors will prescribe DMSO, but only when the patient signs a document acknowledging willingness to assume the responsibility for its use.

How do you find a doctor willing to prescribe and treat a patient with DMSO?

Each doctor has his or her own attitudes and policies with respect to DMSO, and the only sensible thing for a patient to do is to contact a number of doctors to find out their feelings about the drug. Chances are that a doctor who treats you with DMSO will have you sign a form stating that you know you are using a drug for a purpose not expressly approved by the FDA. Veterinarians are a generally good source of DMSO since the DMSO supplied to veterinarians is of a very pure variety.

Is DMSO harmful to the eyes?

The belief that DMSO is harmful to the eyes is based on a more political than scientific decision the FDA made in 1965 to suspend testing on humans because of eye changes that occurred in laboratory animals given large doses of DMSO. Of the eleven animal species that have been tested with DMSO, the changes have been shown to be definite in only three: rabbits, dogs and pigs. There is one study suggesting that these changes are found in monkeys, but four other studies in monkeys refute this finding. There is absolutely no evidence that DMSO causes any adverse eye changes in humans. There has yet to be one documented case of eye damage from DMSO in humans in the nearly two decades that the drug has been used by and tested on humans.

Is it true that DMSO penetrates the skin and goes directly into the system?

Yes. DMSO's ability to penetrate not only the skin but all biological membranes is one of its most unusual properties. Numerous other substances are capable of crossing biological membranes, but with the exception of water, DMSO is in a class by itself among solvents in being able to move in and out of membranes without causing irreversible changes in the membrane structure or in the tissue itself.

What is the safest diluent for DMSO?

Pure water. Some users add a little glycerin, which

keeps the skin from drying, but you should avoid any un-
tried diluents since they may penetrate the skin and produce a measure of systemic toxicity.

*Is it important to inform your doctor that you are using
DMSO?*

Yes, particularly if you are on another medication. One
of the properties of DMSO is to enhance the effect of certain medications a person is taking at the same time. Your
doctor may reduce the dosage of the other medication.

*How can you tell, in the event of an athletic injury, if the
DMSO treatment isn't concealing the presence of a
fracture or a tear?*

Most of the time you can't, which is why you should always take the basic precaution of seeing a doctor or having an X-ray taken with any athletic injury in which there
is even a slight possibility of a break or tear.

Is DMSO better than aspirin for headaches?

Clinical experiments suggest that for certain types of
headaches—sinusitis headaches or headaches caused by
muscular tension in the shoulder and neck—DMSO is an
effective pain reliever, and there is no way of saying
whether it is more or less effective than aspirin. For other
types of headaches—migraine and vascular headaches—
DMSO is much less effective and, in some cases, has been
known to temporarily intensify the pain.

*I've heard that some people gargle with DMSO to relieve
laryngitis. Is this true?*

There have been reports that gargling with DMSO will
relieve the symptoms of laryngitis, but no studies have yet
been done that would compare DMSO's effectiveness
with that of other medications.

Is DMSO good for insect bites and poison ivy?

DMSO is not, generally speaking, effective either for insect bites or for allergic reactions such as those to poison ivy and poison oak. There are a number of dermatitis-like itching conditions for which DMSO can bring prompt relief. Check with your dermatologist.

Does DMSO make you dream more frequently?

Many patients who go on DMSO therapy for any length of time report an increase in the amount of dreaming they do, but the same phenomenon occurs with many medications. In general, DMSO's effect is much milder than that of most prescription drugs.

What is the status of DMSO as a drug in the United States?

As of May, 1981, DMSO was an "approved" drug for only one condition—interstitial cystitis—and in only one concentration: 50 percent. Theoretically, however, a doctor may prescribe this DMSO solution for any condition. Several states now have laws on their books legalizing the manufacture, distribution, sale and use of DMSO within the state. Since these laws may conflict with federal law, the state of Oregon has introduced a special measure in Congress that may result in exempting Oregon from FDA regulations relating to DMSO. Under the Oregon plan, the state would set up its own drug approval system regarding DMSO.

How much will DMSO cost when and if it is approved?

Depending on legislative action, DMSO could cost anywhere from three to fifteen dollars a bottle (wholesale). The price will depend on how much money the company producing the DMSO has had to spend in order to run the tests necessary for approval. In Oregon, should its "memorial" be passed by the Congress, DMSO in an ultra-pure pharmaceutical form will cost about five dollars an eight-ounce bottle. DMSO supplied on a national scale by the pharmaceutical industry could run as high as fifteen dollars, reflecting the costs of the testing needed to gain FDA approval.

How much DMSO should a person use at one time?

Let your doctor determine the proper dosage. For most people, a typical dosage is roughly a tablespoon, although the dosage increases with the size of the area that's being treated. You'll know you're using too much DMSO if it begins to drip off the skin.

How often can a person use DMSO?

Again, let your doctor determine the frequency. Patients being treated for chronic pain conditions usually take DMSO two or three times a day for five days and then go off the substance for two days before resuming it again. For acute conditions (such as a sprained ankle), some trainers recommend more frequent applications of DMSO—as frequently as every two or three hours for the first two or three days after the injury occurs. Some physicians treat acute injuries to the limit of skin tolerance.

Can DMSO give your house a funny odor?

Possibly, yes. People who use large amounts of DMSO and live in houses that have forced-air heating report the odor often permeates the house. One way to reduce this effect is to keep the temperature at as steady a level as possible.

How safe is DMSO?

When used properly and under the supervision of a doctor, DMSO, according to all available scientific evidence at this time, is a safe drug, bearing in mind that no drug is completely safe and that all drugs produce some side effects.

Can DMSO help paraplegics and quadriplegics regain function?

There are many paraplegics and quadriplegics in the United States who have been on DMSO therapy for months and even years. Some have recovered certain functions no one thought they would ever recover. Whether this function would have returned even without DMSO cannot be proven. Only a few controlled studies on humans are being conducted at this time, and these concentrate on head injuries. Laboratory studies, as well as a handful of clinical cases, suggest that if DMSO is introduced systemically immediately following a serious spinal-cord or head injury (within one hour in spinal-cord injuries; within six hours in head injuries), patients who might otherwise be dead or paralyzed for life can survive and even be spared the paralysis such injury could otherwise bring about.

How does DMSO interact with alcohol?

The interrelationship between DMSO and alcohol is poorly understood. Some studies show that if the two substances are ingested at the same time, DMSO will accelerate the normal effects of alcohol in the body. Otherwise, the effects are much less pronounced. In general, patients on DMSO therapy are advised to use alcohol conservatively.

What are DMSO's main side effects?

The most commonly reported side effects of DMSO are: (1) a slight redness or itching at the site of application; (2) a garlic or oyster-like taste in the mouth; (3) an unpleasant breath odor. Newer formulations of DMSO, available only in Oregon at the present time, have served to minimize these effects. In rare cases, a patient may develop a generalized body rash.

What is the best way to counteract the itching and the rash that sometimes develop when a person uses DMSO?

If the rash is severe, DMSO treatment should be stopped immediately or else the solution should be weakened by adding water. For milder reactions, any of the over-the-counter lower-level corticosteroid creams and lotions should relieve the itching and the redness. Sometimes cornstarch is effective. Consult your doctor.

What basic precautions should a person taking DMSO follow?

Your doctor is the best judge. Because DMSO has the capacity to carry other substances with it, across the skin barrier and into the system, most doctors will advise you to avoid direct contact to the application area of any other, possibly toxic, material, such as insecticide. Some physicians also caution against bringing into immediate contact with the application area any clothing made of synthetic material. This caution is well advised with fabrics and ornaments made of acrylic, rayon, and some other synthetics, since DMSO may dissolve these materials. Fabrics made of wool, cotton, nylon or polyester are unaffected by DMSO.

What causes the bad breath and the funny taste of DMSO?

The most plausible explanation for the bad breath and funny taste that often accompany DMSO use is that DMSO enhances whatever odors or tastes may already be inside your body. Pure DMS (dimethyl sulfide), one of the two metabolites of DMSO, has a reasonably pleasant, ether-like odor, but it enhances both good smells—such as perfumes—and bad smells, People who have bad breath to begin with will find that DMSO increases it.

Is there anything that can be done to cut the taste and odor caused by DMSO?

Nor much, unfortunately. Chewing gum, brushing your teeth or taking breath sweeteners is only of temporary help. Newly developed DMSO products, however, have reduced to a minimum the breath, aftertaste, and skin itching and irritation experienced with DMSO.

What does "approved drug" mean?

The National Academy of Sciences, in a DMSO report submitted to the FDA in 1972, describes the meaning of "approved drug" as follows:

> No new drug may be introduced into interstate commerce in the United States unless it has been approved by the Food and Drug Administration. Under the Federal Food, Drug, and Cosmetic Act (21 USC 355), the Commissioner of Food and Drugs may not approve a new drug if adequate tests show that it is unsafe for the use proposed, or if tests do not show that it *is* safe. And the Commissioner may not approve a new drug if available information to him shows that there is a lack of substantial evidence that the drug will have the effect it is represented to have.

What is the drug approval process in the United States?

Before a drug can be approved by the FDA, the manufacturer or investigator behind the drug must first submit something known as an IND, a Notice of Claimed Investigational Exemption for a New Drug. This exemption allows a manufacturer to conduct clinical investigations necessary before the submission of something known as an NDA, or New Drug Application. The FDA, by virtue of the powers given it in the Federal Food, Drug, and Cosmetic Act, can refuse to approve a New Drug Application for any of the following reasons:

1. When the results of tests show that the drug is unsafe for use under the conditions prescribed, recommended, or suggested in the proposed labeling, or else fail to show that the drug is safe.

2. If, "upon the basis of any other information before him [not submitted by the applicant], he [the commissioner] has insufficient information to determine whether such drug is safe for use under such conditions."

3. If, when "evaluated on the basis of the information submitted to him as part of the application and any other information before him with respect to such drug, there is a lack of substantial evidence that it will have the effect it purports or is represented to have under the conditions of use prescribed, recommended, or suggested in the proposed labelling thereof."

Bibliography

Ashwood-Smith, M. J. "Radioprotective and Cryoprotective Properties of Dimethyl Sulfoxide in Cellular Systems." *Annals of the New York Academy of Sciences,* Vol. 141 (1967), p. 45.

Berliner, D. L., and A. G. Ruhrman. "The Influence of Dimethyl Sulfoxide on Fibroblastic Proliferation." *Annals of the New York Academy of Sciences,* Vol. 141 (1967), p. 159.

Blumenthal, L. S., and M. Fuchs. "The Clinical Use of Dimethyl Sulfoxide on Various Headaches, Musculoskeletal and Other General Medical Disorders." *Annals of the New York Academy of Sciences,* Vol. 141 (1967), p. 572.

Brobyn, R. B. "The Human Toxicology of Dimethyl Sulfoxide." *Annals of the New York Academy of Sciences,* Vol. 243 (1975), p. 497.

Brown, J. H. "A Double-Blind Clinical Study—DMSO for Acute Injuries and Inflammation Compared to Accepted Therapy." *Current Therapeutic Research,* Vol. 13 (1971), p. 536.

Brown, J. Harold. "Clinical Experience With DMSO in Acute Musculoskeletal Conditions, Comparing a Noncontrolled Series With a Controlled Double Blind Study." *Annals of the New York Academy of Sciences,* Vol. 141 (1967), p. 496.

Brown, V. K., J. Robinson, and D. E. Stevenson. "A Note on the Toxicity and Solvent Properties of Dimethyl Sulfoxide." *Journal of Pharmacy and Pharmacology,* Vol. 15 (1963), p. 688.

Cortese, T. A. "DMSO in Dermatology." *Dimehyl Sulfoxide,* Vol. 1, *Basic Concepts,* eds. S. W. Jacob et al. New York: Marcel Dekker, Inc., 1971, p. 337.

Day, P. L. "DMSO Evaluation With Approximately 1000 Patients in the Orthopedic Practice." Study presented at Biological Actions of DMSO Symposium, ed. A. G. Schering. University of Vienna, 1966.

de La Torre, J. C. *The Spinal Cord and Its Reaction to Traumatic Injury,* ed. W. F. Windle. Marcel Dekker, Inc. New York: 1980.

——, and P. K. Hill. *Dynamics of Brain Edema.* Berlin: Springer-Verlag, 1976, pp. 306–314.

de La Torre, J. C., et al. "Modifications of Experimental Spinal Cord Injuries Using Dimethyl Sulfoxide." *Transactions of the American Neurological Association,* Vol. 97 (1971), p. 230.

de La Torre, J. C., et al. "Dimethyl Sulfoxide in the Treatment of Experimental Brain Compression." *Journal of Neurosurgery,* Vol. 38 (1972), p. 343.

de La Torre, J. C., et al. "Dimethylsulfoxide in Central Nervous System Trauma." *Annals of the New York Academy of Sciences,* Vol. 243 (1975), p. 362.

Demos, C. H., et al. "Dimethyl Sulfoxide in Musculoskeletal Disorders." *Annals of the New York Academy of Sciences,* Vol. 141 (1967), p. 517.

Dujovny, M., et al. "The Role of DMSO and Methylprednisolone in Canine Middle Cerebral Artery Microsurgical Embolectomy." *Stroke,* Vol. 8, No. 1 (1977).

Ehrlich, G. E., and R. Joseph. "Dimethyl Sulfoxide in Scleraderma." *Pennsylvania Medical Journal,* Vol. 68 (1965), p. 51.

Engel, M. F. "Indications and Contraindications for the Use of DMSO in Clinical Dermatology." *Annals of the New York Academy of Sciences,* Vol. 141 (1967), p. 638.

——. "Dimethylsulfoxide in the Treatment of Scleroderma." *Southern Medical Journal,* Vol. 65, No. 1 (1972), p. 71.

Feldman, W. E., J. D. Punch, and P. C. Holden. "In Vivo and in Vitro Effects of Dimethyl Sulfoxide on Streptomycin-Sensitive and Resistant Escherichia Coli." *Annals of the New York Academy of Sciences*, Vol. 243 (1975), p. 269.

Finney, J. W., et al. "Protection of the Ischemic Heart With DMSO Alone or DMSO With Hydrogen Peroxide." *Annals of the New York Academy of Sciences*, Vol. 141 (1967), p. 231.

Franz, T. J., and J. J. Van Bruggen. "A Possible Mechanism of Action of DMSO." *Annals of the New York Academy of Sciences*, Vol. 141 (1967), p. 302.

Frommhold, W., C. Bublitz, and G. Gries. "The Use of DMSO for the Treatment of Postirradiation Subcutaneous Plaques." *Annals of the New York Academy of Sciences*, Vol. 141 (1967), p. 603.

Gerhards, E., and H. Cibian. "The Metabolism of Dimethyl Sulfoxide and Its Metabolic Effects in Man and Animals." *Annals of the New York Academy of Sciences*, Vol. 141 (1967), p. 65.

Gorog, P., and I. B. Kovacs. "Effects of Topically Applied Dimethyl Sulfoxide." *Annals of the New York Academy of Sciences*, Vol. 243 (1975), p. 91.

Hagglund, E. K. M., and T. U. E. Enkvist. *Method of Improving the Yield of Methyl Sulfide Obtained by Heating Waste Liquors From Cellulose Manufacture by Adding Inorganic Sulfides.* U.S. Patent Office No. 2,711,430, Washington, D.C., June 21, 1955.

Haigler, H. J., and D. D. Spring. "Dimethyl Sulfoxide (DMSO): Analgesic Effects in Rats." *Federation Proceedings*, Vol. 40, No. 288 (1981), p. 285.

Herschler, R. J., and S. W. Jacob. "A New Drug From Lignin." *TAPPI*, Vol. 48 (1965), p. 43.

Jacob, S. W. "Dimethyl Sulfoxide, Its Basic Pharmacology and Usefulness in the Therapy of Headache." *Headache*, Vol. 5, No. 78 (1965), p. 414.

——, and D. C. Wood. "Dimethyl Sulfoxide (DMSO): Toxicology, Pharmacology and Clinical Experience." *American Journal of Surgery*, Vol. 114 (1967), p. 414.

——, M. Bischel, and R. J. Herschler. "Dimethyl Sulfoxide (DMSO), a New Concept in Pharmacotherapy." *Current Therapeutic Research*, Vol. 6 (1964), p. 134.

——, M. Bischel, and R. J. Herschler. "Dimethylsulfoxide: Effects on the Permeability of Biologic Membranes (Preliminary Report)." *Current Therapeutic Research*, Vol. 6 (1964), p. 193.

——, E. R. Rosenbaum, and D. C. Wood. *Dimethyl Sulfoxide*, Vol. 1, *Basic Concepts*. New York: Marcel Dekker, Inc., 1971.

——, et al. "The Influence of Dimethylsulfoxide on the Transport of Insulin Across a Biologic Membrane." *Federation Proceedings*, Vol. 23 (1964), p. 410.

Jacob, S. W., ed. "DMSO-Dimethyl Sulfoxide." *Dimethyl Sulfoxide*, Vol. 1, *Basic Concepts*, New York: Marcel Dekker, Inc., 1971.

John, H. "Therapeutische Erfahrungen mit Dimethylsulfoxyd in der orthopädischen Praxis." *Arzneim. Forsch.*, Vol. 15 (1965), p. 1298.

John, H., and G. Laudahn. "Clinical Experiences With the Topical Application of DMSO in Orthopedic Diseases: Evaluation of 4180 Cases." *Annals of the New York Academy of Sciences*, Vol. 141 (1967), p. 506.

Juel-Jensen, B. E., et al. "Treatment of Zoster With Idoxuridine in Dimethyl Sulphoxide." *British Medical Journal*, Vol. 4 (1970), p. 776.

Kappert, A. "Experimental and Clinical Evaluation of Topical Dimethyl Sulfoxide in Venous Disorders of the Extremities." *Annals of the New York Academy of Sciences*, Vol. 243 (1975), p. 403.

Katz, R., and R. W. Hood. "Topical Thiabendazole for Creeping Eruption." *Archives of Dermatology*, Vol. 94 (1966), p. 643.

Kocsis, J. J., S. Harkaway, and R. Snyder. "Biological Effects of the Metabolites of Dimethyl Sulfoxide." *Annals of the New York Academy of Sciences*, Vol. 243 (1975), p. 104.

Kolb, K. H., et al. "Absorption, Distribution and Elimination of Labeled Dimethyl Sulfoxide in Man and Animals." *Annals of the New York Academy of Sciences*, Vol. 141 (1967), p. 85.

Kunze, M. "Production of Interferon in the White Mouse by Dimethyl Sulfoxide." *Annals of the New York Academy of Sciences*, Vol. 243 (1975), p. 308.

Lackey, H. B., S. W. Jacob, and R. J. Herschler. *Purification of Dialkyl Sulfoxides*. Belgian Patent No. 656, 879, June 9, 1965.

Lim, R., and S. Mullan. "Enhancement of Resistance of Glial Cells by Dimethyl Sulfoxide Against Sonic Disruption." *Annals of the New York Academy of Sciences*, Vol. 243 (1975), p. 358.

Lockie, L. M., and B. M. Norcross. "A Clinical Study on the Effects of Dimethyl Sulfoxide in 103 Patients With Acute and Chronic Musculoskeletal Injuries and Inflammations." *Annals of the New York Academy of Sciences*, Vol. 141 (1967), p. 599.

Mallach, H. J. "Interaction of DMSO and Alcohol." *Annals of the New York Academy of Sciences*, Vol. 141 (1967), p. 457.

Martin, D., and H. G. Hauthal. *Dimethyl Sulfoxide*. New York: John Wiley & Sons, Halsted Press, 1975.

Matsumoto, J. "Clinical Trials of Dimethyl Sulfoxide in Rheumatoid Arthritis Patients in Japan." *Annals of the New York Academy of Sciences*, Vol. 141 (1967) p. 560.

National Academy of Sciences—National Research Council. *Dimethyl Sulfoxide as a Therapeutic Agent*. Contract FDA 70-22, Task Order No. 14, 1974.

Ogden, H. D. "Experiences With DMSO in Treatment for Headache." *Annals of the New York Academy of Sciences*, Vol. 141 (1967) p. 646.

Parsons, J. L., W. L. Shepard, and W. M. Fosdick. "DMSO as an Adjuvant to Physical Therapy in the Chronic Frozen Shoulder." *Annals of the New York Academy of Sciences*, Vol. 141 (1967), p. 569.

Paul, M. M. "Interval Therapy With Dimethyl Sulfoxide."

Annals of the New York Academy of Sciences, Vol. 141 (1967), p. 586.

Penrod, D. S., B. Bacharach, and J. Y. Templeton. "Dimethyl Sulfoxide for Incisional Pain After Thoracotomy, Preliminary Report." *Annals of the New York Academy of Sciences*, Vol. 141 (1967), p. 493.

Persky, L., and B. H. Stewart. "The Use of Dimethyl Sulfoxide in the Treatment of Genitourinary Disorders." *Annals of the New York Academy of Sciences*, Vol. 141 (1967), p. 551.

Peterson, C. G., and R. D. Robertson. "A Pharmacodynamic Study of Dimethyl Sulfoxide." *Annals of the New York Academy of Sciences*, Vol. 141 (1967), p. 273.

Rosenbaum, W. M., E. E. Rosenbaum, and S. W. Jacob. "The Use of Dimethyl Sulfoxide (DMSO) for the Treatment of Intractable Pain of Surgical Patients." *Surgery*, Vol. 58 (1965), p. 258.

Rubin, L. F., and F. A. Mattis. "Dimethylsulfoxide: Lens Changes in Dogs During Oral Administration." *Science*, Vol. 153 (1966), p. 83.

Sams, Jr., W. M. "The Effects of Dimethyl Sulfoxide on Nerve Conduction." *Annals of the New York Academy of Sciences*, Vol. 141 (1967), p. 242.

Scherbel, A. L. "Further Observations on the Effect of DMSO on Patients With Generalized Scleroderma." Study presented at Biological Actions of DMSO Symposium, ed. A. G. Schering, University of Vienna, 1966.

——, L. J. McCormack, and M. J. Poppo. "Alteration of Collagen in Generalized Scleroderma After Treatment With Dimethylsulfoxide." *Cleveland Clinic Quarterly*, Vol. 32 (1965), p. 47.

——, L. J. McCormack, and J. K. Layle. "Further Observations on the Effect of Dimethyl Sulfoxide in Patients With Generalized Scleroderma." *Annals of the New York Academy of Sciences*, Vol. 141 (1967), p. 613.

Seibert, F. B., F. K. Farrelly, and C. C. Shephard. "DMSO and Other Combatants Against Bacteria Isolated From Leukemia and Cancer Patients." *Annals of the New York Academy of Sciences*, Vol. 141 (1967), p. 175.

Sergayev, V. P., and R. Z. Zakiev. "Treatment of Scleroderma With Dimethyl Sulfoxide." *Vestnik Dermatologii i Venerologii*, Vol. 3 (1976), p. 70.

Shealy, C. N. "The Physiological Substrate of Pain." *Headache*, Vol. 6 (1966), p. 101.

Shlafer, M., and A. M. Karow, Jr. "Pharmacological Effects of Dimethyl Sulfoxide on the Mammalian Myocardium." *Annals of the New York Academy of Sciences*, Vol. 243 (1975), p. 110.

Smith, G. C. "Observations in Treating Cutaneous Larva Migrans." *Journal South Carolina Medical Association*, Vol. 62 (1966), p. 265.

Sommer, S., and G. Tauberger. "Toxicologic Investigations of Dimethyl Sulfoxide." *Arzneim. Forsch.*, Vol. 14 (1964), p. 1050.

Steinberg, A. "The Employment of Dimethyl Sulfoxide as an Anti-Inflammatory Agent and Steroid-Transporter in Diversified Clinical Diseases." *Annals of the New York Academy of Sciences*, Vol. 141 (1967), p. 532.

Stewart, B. H., et al. "The Treatment of Patients With Special Reference to Intravesical DMSO." *Journal of Urology*, Vol. 107 (1972), p. 377.

Stewart, B. H., and S. W. Shirley. "Further Experience With Intravesical Dimethyl Sulfoxide in Treatment of Interstitial Cystitis." *Journal of Urology*, Vol. 116 (1976), p. 36.

Tuffanelli, D. L. "A Clinical Trial With Dimethylsulfoxide in Scleroderma." *Archives of Dermatology*, Vol. 93 (1966), p. 724.

Waller, F. T., et al. "DMSO for Reduction of Intracranial Pressure." Abstract in *Journal of Neurosurgery*, September, 1979.

Ward, J. R., M. L. Miller, and S. Marcus. "The Effect of Dimethyl Sulfoxide on the Local Schwartzman Phenomena." *Annals of the New York Academy of Sciences*, Vol. 141 (1967), p. 280.

Warren, J., et al. "Potentiation of Antineoplastic Compounds by Oral Dimethyl Sulfoxide in Tumor-Bearing Rats." *Annals of the New York Academy of Sciences*, Vol. 243 (1975), p. 194.

Weissman, G., G. Sessa, and V. Bevans. "Effect of DMSO on the Stabilization of Lyosomes by Cortisone and Chloroquine in Vitro." *Annals of the New York Academy of Sciences*, Vol. 141 (1967), p. 326.

Williams, K. I., S. H. Burstein, and D. S. Layne. "Dimethyl Sulfone-Isolated From Human Urine." *Archives of Biochemistry and Biophysics*, Vol. 113 (1966), p. 251.

Willson, J. E., D. E. Brown, and E. K. Timmens. "A Toxicological Study of Dimethylsulfoxide." *Toxicology and Applied Pharmacology*, Vol. 7 (1965), p. 104.

Yorio, T., and P. J. Bentley. "The Effects of Hyperosmotic Agents on the Electrical Properties of the Amphibian Lens in Vitro." *Experimental Eye Research*, Vol. 22, No. 3 (1976), p. 195.

Zuckner, J., J. Uddin, and George E. Gantner, Jr. "Local Application of Dimethyl Sulfoxide and DMSO Combined With Triamcinolone Acetonide in Rheumatoid Arthritis." *Annals of the New York Academy of Sciences*, Vol. 141 (1967), p. 555.

Appendix I

Among the legions of DMSO advocates throughout the United States are prominent physicians, scientists and elected officials. What follows are some of the statements that have been issued by some of these people at different periods throughout the controversy.

Rep. Mary Rose Oakar, D., Ohio
Testimony given before the Select Committee on Aging, House of Representatives, March 24, 1980.

First of all, I want to commend you for having this hearing. I want to congratulate my friend, Congressman Duncan, for being here. He is well known as one of the fairest people and nicest people in Congress as well as the most knowledgeable.

Bob, I think you are being a little kind with respect to the FDA, if you don't mind my saying so. There are many cases, in my judgment and based on the limited research that we have done here, in which the FDA was extraordinarily scrupulous when it came to releasing drugs for use by the American people, and not at all cautious in other cases.

We just heard, for example, that they whisked a drug to Yugoslavia for Chairman Tito who is dying, and yet our own people who are dying with the same kind of affliction cannot get this so-called miracle drug.

We know that a Federal Jury recently awarded $20,000 in damages to parents of a child born with birth defects caused by Bendectin, a drug commonly used for morning sickness during the first three months of pregnancy. Medical journals have reported 180 cases of birth defects due to Bendectin, and yet this drug has not been questioned at all by the FDA or taken off the market.

We know that even aspirin, which is frequently prescribed for arthritis and other types of afflictions, can be damaging. I want to ask some questions, when we get to some of the doctors, about aspirin and other drugs, and also whether they are being unmercifully scrupulous to a point of absurdity when it comes to DMSO. While I will accept, as a Member of Congress, some of the responsibility for some of their scrupulosity, I will not accept all of it because I think they have hindered progress in many areas.

Rep. Robert Duncan, D., Oregon
Testimony given before the Senate Health and Scientific Research Sub-committee, July 31, 1980.

I was influential in setting up one of the first meetings with the FDA and getting the DMSO tests lined up to see whether it was efficacious to meet the standards. The subject matter was scleroderma and the question was whether DMSO could bring relief for scleroderma in the extremities. There was no other relief for the ulcers in the fingertips that some scleroderma patients get except, on occasion, amputation of the fingers. Now, here we are some sixteen years later after that first meeting with scleroderma still not approved as a disease for which DMSO can be used.

There has been some progress made. I want this committee to know that I am sympathetic with the problems that the FDA has in operating under a law which we ourselves passed and which requires them to find this drug not only efficacious but safe, and I am concerned about the standards of proof that are set up by the FDA in order to permit a drug like this to go on the market.

I know they have a narrow line to tread between letting a thalidomide on the market, for instance, and keeping something like DMSO off. I am sympathetic to them.

I thought as I drove in here this morning that we will have serious impact on men's fortunes by a standard of proof which we call a preponderance of the evidence. We will even deprive people of their liberty by a standard called "beyond a reasonable doubt."

But it seems to me that for drugs, and particularly for DMSO, we are demanding a standard of proof that is almost unattainable. In all of these years of use, can we say there are no side effects? No, there is no free lunch in this country. But the side effects are so minimal that one could almost say there are none.

With respect to my own use of it, the most serious side effect is a threatened divorce by my wife because she doesn't like the odor. Dr. Jacob has removed some of the odor and he has masked it in another preparation by a wintergreen flavor.

I asked my wife if she didn't like the wintergreen flavor, and if that wouldn't remove her objections. She said, no. Instead of smelling like the tidal flats at Bayonne, New Jersey, when the tide is out, she said you now smell like the locker room of the Green Bay Packers. But that odor is infinitesimal compared with the relief.

But the drug has been shown to have good results in so many instances and the people who have used it are so enthusiastic that the scientists downtown naturally, I think, get suspicious about it.

Somebody asked me what it was good for the other day and I said, did your mother give you medicine when you were a kid and you asked what is this for, and she said, take it, it is good for what ails you.

I think I first got a hold of it for my horses. It was good for my horses. It is approved for use in most of Western Europe, the Soviet Union, a lot of countries in South and Central America and in Japan. I obtained some of it from sailor friends of mine from Japan.

I have observed its beneficial effects for arthritis, bursitis, the reduction of swelling and inflammation. I have seen it almost make shingles disappear like a miracle. I have watched it in serious burns on myself and I watched the pain go away in a matter of minutes. I saw that the serious burn barely got pink and never swelled blisters. Dr. Jacob will tell you about these things. With your permission. I will ask you to put my prepared statement in the record.

Dr. Arthur Scherbel, Chief of Rheumatology, Cleveland Clinic Foundation

Testimony given before the Select Committee on Aging, House of Representatives, March 24, 1980.

Indeed, I would want DMSO among the drugs that I use commonly in the treatment of pain. Frequently, one cannot give one drug to a patient and get an excellent relief of pain in the diseases that we were talking about. Arthritis is not simple. If a patient with arthritis improves quickly while taking some simple drug, my impression is that the arthritis was not serious. I am talking about the serious illnesses, progressive arthritis or scleroderma with persistent ulcers, or impending amputation.

The controversy that exists over the clinical effectiveness of DMSO is not well founded—clinical effectiveness may be variable in different patients. If toxicity is consistently minimal, the drug should not be restricted from use in clinical practice. It is my opinion that the clinical effectiveness of DMSO can be decided with complete satisfaction if the drug is made available to the practicing physician. The number of patient complaints about pain and the number of phone calls to the doctor's office will decide quickly whether or not the drug is effective."

Senator Edward Kennedy, D., Massachusetts
Testimony given before the Senate Health and Scientific Research Sub-committee, July 31, 1980.

Today, the Senate Health Subcommittee will hear the story of DMSO. It is a sad story, sad because hundreds of thousands of Americans suffering from a variety of painful and often disabling diseases have placed their hopes in this drug, and yet after eighteen years we still do not know whether or not those hopes are misplaced. It is a story of failure—failure of the bureaucracy at the Food and Drug Administration to handle the drug appropriately, to expedite a complete and timely review, to detect serious deficiencies in scientific data submitted on the drug's behalf, to satisfy the public that it is doing all it can to develop definitive answers; failure of the private sector to conduct competent and acceptable scientific research on the drug, to adequately monitor the quality of work being done, and to cooperate fully with the FDA investigations of possible wrongdoing. This failure of both federal and industrial responsibility has had a very high cost: the erosion of public confidence in the ability of government—in this case, the FDA—to work, to respond to human suffering, to meet people's needs.

As a result, over 100,000 Americans use DMSO each year. They get it however they can: in some cases legally, in some cases not; in some cases in forms designed for human use, in some cases not. A tiny minority of these people use DMSO for its one legitimately approved purpose, but in most cases they use it for unapproved purposes. Some rub it on their skin; some drink it; some are treated intravenously. By the tens of thousands, Americans are making individual judgments to try DMSO for arthritis, for ankle sprains, for neurological trauma and for a variety of other reasons. Others are desperate to try it. And many of those who use it believe that they are helped, and tell their friends, and the use of the drug spreads. We will hear some of these case histories this morning, and they are impressive.

But it is important to remember that the proper place to evaluate the safety and effectiveness of a new drug is in the Food and Drug Administration, not the news media. The proper way to evaluate it is by scientific, medical trials conducted by the drug company, not by individual subjective judgments. This nation has always insisted, and rightly so, that a drug be proven safe and effective before it is marketed. This safeguard has spared the nation the thalidomide-like tragedies. And yet a very fine balance must be maintained by the Food and Drug Administration, for as tragic as it may be to let an unsafe drug on the market, it may be equally tragic to keep breakthrough drugs off the market . . . drugs which may save lives, restore normal functioning, or alleviate unbearable pain.

To maintain that balance requires public confidence in both the ability of the FDA to make approval or nonapproval decisions rapidly and the ability of private industry to conduct competent and scientific studies. That confidence has not been earned with DMSO. Its eighteen-year odyssey has made a travesty of the regulatory process.

I do not know if DMSO works or not, but with the hopes of so many Americans riding on it, with so many others already using it, I believe a definitive evaluation must be made, and made soon. Therefore, I have directed that the staff of the subcommittee convene a meeting as soon as possible among the FDA, the NIH, and all the manufacturers interested in marketing this product. The purpose would be to determine what needs to be done, and to develop a timetable for doing it. I cannot promise those Americans who look to DMSO to cure their ills that it will turn out to be a wonder drug, but I can and do promise to end the wondering about it and replace it with some definitive answers.

Rep. Steven D. Symms, R., Idaho
Testimony given before the Senate Health and Research Sub-committee, July 31, 1980.

I think, as mentioned, that many of us are grateful to the FDA for the work they did to stop thalidomide from being sold in the United States. On the other hand, the nature of bureaucrats is to say no rather than say yes because when they say yes, they do have to take some risks. When they say no, then they are not taking any risks and there are no responsibilities or disruptions that may come. So this is what we are dealing with.

I would just say, Mr. Chairman, to you and members of the Committee, I consider it a privilege to be here today and to testify on the innovation and availability of DMSO in the United States and, further-more, I again would like to commend you for having these hearings so that maybe we can get this important subject off dead center.

As you on the Committee know, I have introduced three bills in the House in conjunction with Congressman Bob Duncan which would approve the usage of DMSO for the treatment of scleroderma, for the treatment of arthritis, bursitis, rheumatism and other disorders of the muscular-skeletal system, and approve the intravenous use of DMSO for the treatment of acute brain and spinal-cord injuries.

Normally, I do not like to introduce legislation for the approval of specific drugs because I believe that the entire process by which the Food and Drug Administration approves drugs for use in the United States should be revamped, and in this regard I have a major reform bill pending in the House, the Food and Drug Reform Act of 1979, which is commonly called H.R. 54, dealing with a broad range of the problems, some of which have already been discussed this morning, the efficacy question, the patent question, and some of the things I think would help move ahead our protection and our safety but also expedite the use of vital pharmaceutical drugs that we need.

I think that I have said many times that there is nothing more ineffective than a product that is unavailable to the public. I think that that is where we have been too carried away with our entire attitude toward efficacy.

However, Mr. Chairman, because DMSO can provide widespread relief for those suffering from muscular-skeletal disorders such as arthritis; provide treatment to those suffering from scleroderma, a disabling disorder in which the skin becomes tight, interfering with blood supply and joint movement; and oftentimes save the lives of those patients who are suffering from injuries or hemorrhaging within the brain because of the ability to reduce intracranial pressure, I believed that specific legislation was urgently needed to make DMSO available for prescriptive use in the United States.

Despite a myriad of tests and a multitude of patients testifying to the safety and efficacy of DMSO, the Food and Drug Administration still enforces its go-slow edict on DMSO. As a result of the time and money that it would take to encourage the FDA to get this compound onto the market, many researchers and pharmacological companies have backed off in their studies.

There is very little that can be said in a complimentary vein for the FDA, for it has been a tremendous obstacle to the progress of medicine. The FDA has been solely responsible for driving modern medical research out of this country to foreign soil. Unfortunately, the attitude that more regulations and prohibitions will insure the safety of the citizens of the United States is totally distorted. The fact of the matter is that FDA constraints have caused undue suffering and the loss of life and limb to many of the citizens here in the United States.

Appendix II

U.S. SENATE HEARINGS
SUB-COMMITTEE ON HEALTH
Washington, D. C.
July 31, 1980

Statement by Stanley W. Jacob, M.D.

The passage of the Kefauver-Harris amendments in 1962 has been followed by an obvious drug lag in the United States. By "drug lag" I mean:

Reduced rate of discovery and development of new therapeutic entities.

Increased period of time to move new drug discoveries from the laboratory to prescriptive use.

Restricted release of new drug entities in the United States compared with other technically advanced countries.

Since 1962, the United States Food and Drug Administration has grown in both power and population—in many ways like a malignant tumor. There are at least four serious side effects secondary to the way the FDA has functioned:

FDA regulations have increased the cost for therapeutic substances.

FDA regulations have brought about a termination of research on many therapeutants which might be useful in so-called "orphan" diseases, i.e., diseases affecting fewer than 100,000 Americans.

FDA regulations have brought about a de-emphasis on research and development of the so-called "soft" (less toxic) drugs which are difficult or impossible to clear through the present methodology of efficacy required by the FDA. If aspirin were to be introduced today, it would fall into the category of a "soft" agent of low toxicity.

The FDA has brought about a de-emphasis of research and development on drug combinations.

I would like to discuss dimethyl sulfoxide (DMSO).

My major research interest since 1962 has been the pharmacology and clinical usefulness of DMSO.

Dimethyl sulfoxide in the United States is derived from lignin, the cement substance of trees. It can, however, be made from a number of organic chemicals and may be inexpensively produced.

DMSO was first chemically prepared in 1866 but remained a laboratory curiosity for more than three quarters of a century. In 1948, a number of papers began to appear in the chemical literature showing it was a solvent for many other substances. In 1959, a group in Great Britain demonstrated that dimethyl sulfoxide would protect red blood cells and other tissues against freezing damage.

The use of DMSO as a drug was not shown until a collaborative effort between scientists at the University of Oregon Medical School and the Crown Zellerbach Corp. demonstrated in laboratory tests that DMSO would not only pass through the skin and mucous membranes, but during passage would carry with it a certain number of other substances. For instance, penicillin can be dissolved in DMSO and be carried through the skin without a needle.

In these early studies, dimethyl sulfoxide was shown to relieve pain, reduce swelling, slow the growth of bacteria, improve blood supply, soften scar tissue, enhance the effectiveness of other pharmacologic agents, serve as a diuretic, and act as a muscle relaxant.

The first report on the use of dimethyl sulfoxide as a pharmacologic agent was written in 1963 and published February 1, 1964. The first IND to study DMSO clinically in the United States was submitted on October 25, 1963. Three NDA's on DMSO were submitted to the FDA in 1965. All were turned down. A fourth NDA was submitted in 1970. It was also turned down by the FDA.

Yet, *The New York Times* in a lead editorial on April 3, 1965, called DMSO "the closest thing to a wonder drug produced in the 1960's."

Several thousand scientific articles on DMSO have appeared in the world's literature. In our reference library at the University of Oregon Health Sciences Center, we have a fairly complete bibliography which includes seven technical books on dimethyl sulfoxide.

Four international symposia have been held on DMSO. The first of these was in Berlin, Germany, in July, 1965. The second was under the auspices of the New York Academy of Sciences in March of 1966, New York City, New York. The third was sponsored by the University of Vienna, in Austria, November, 1966. The fourth was again in New York, under the sponsorship of the New York Academy of Sciences in January, 1974.

Of major importance is the fact that DMSO has been shown to be of value, not only in diseases for which there is other known treatment, but in a number of illnesses for which no other effective or low-risk treatment is known, such as the painful ulcers of the fingers in patients with scleroderma. In this disease the skin becomes tight and the joints are prevented from moving. Microscopic sections of skin from patients with scleroderma have been studied before and after treatment of DMSO. These studies demonstrated definite improvements with DMSO therapy—without DMSO, some of these patients would require amputations.

The value of DMSO in other illnesses for which effective pharmacologic treatment does not presently exist, includes severe abacterial prostatitis, Dupuytren's contracture, subcutaneous scarring from cobalt irradiation, keloids, Peyronie's disease and potentially in otherwise "irreversible" injury to the brain and spinal cord.

A broader spectrum of primary pharmacology and clinical benefit, both actual and potential, has been described in the scientific literature for DMSO than for any other substance with which I am familiar. No attempt will be made at this point to record the long list of entities for which benefit from DMSO has already been responsibly reported in the literature. In my opinion, DMSO is the treatment of choice for severe acute musculoskeletal trauma (such as strains and sprains) and acute and chronic bursitis.

Dimethyl sulfoxide is a useful adjunct in the treatment of rheumatoid arthritis, degenerative arthritis and gouty arthritis. It primarily will relieve pain, but will also reduce inflammation and increase joint mobility. Due to its effectiveness in the treatment of arthritis, Americans by the thousands are flocking to nations such as Mexico to receive DMSO. In Mexico they are charged seven to eight hundred dollars for three days of treatment. One entrepreneur in this "South of the Border" country presumably treated with DMSO thirty thousand Americans last year for arthritis and grossed over twenty million dollars.

The effectiveness of DMSO has been demonstrated by

comparative studies, by "double blind" studies, and by the clinical impression type of evaluations in man.

Dr. J. Harold Brown, formerly President of the Aerospace Medical Association, included in this "double blind" report the following statement:

> "I am convinced that topical application of DMSO in the treatment of acute musculoskeletal conditions is a striking and significant therapeutic contribution. During the period of time I conducted clinical investigation with this medication, I practically discarded physical therapy as treatment for musculoskeletal problems because the rehabilitation of my patients was so prompt with DMSO. There was little or no necessity to prescribe narcotics and tranquilizers since pain was promptly mitigated following topical application of DMSO."

The further usefulness of DMSO has been shown by the fact that it is now prescriptive in the United States for acute musculoskeltal problems in small and large animals, approved by the Veterinary Division of the Food and Drug Administration in 1970.

An important question about any drug is toxicity. There is no such thing as a non-toxic drug. DMSO has its side effects. The major side effect of DMSO is the possibility of an occasional patient being hypersensitive.

I believe there are more data on animal toxicology regarding DMSO than have ever existed for any other experimental drug. I have not had experience with any drug in medicine which I consider to be safer. In my estimation there are more data on human toxicology of DMSO than have ever been obtained for any other experimental drug. The Food and Drug Administration itself has data on over one hundred thousand patients. Despite the prescriptive use of DMSO worldwide, there is, to my knowledge, not a single case of well-documented serious toxicity.

Dimethyl sulfoxide is currently a prescriptive agent in the United States for interstitial cystitis. It is prescriptive in Canada for scleroderma. It is prescriptive in Great Britain and Ireland for shingles when mixed with IDU. It is prescriptive for a whole range of disorders for topical administration in Germany, Austria, and Switzerland. It is widely prescriptive in many parts of South America. It is prescriptive in the Soviet Union and has been since 1971.

When Dr. Chauncy Leake, one of the world's most eminent pharmacologists, reviewed the New York Academy of Sciences Symposium on DMSO in 1966, he stated that the well known legal phrase *res ipsa loquitur* applied to the DMSO situation. In summarizing the conference, Dr. Leake said,

> "Rarely had a new drug come to the attention of the scientific community with so much verifiable information, from so many parts of the world, both as to safety and effectiveness."

There is little doubt but that DMSO should be prescriptive in the United States today for a whole host of disorders, including its potential for pain relief in arthritis. It is prescriptive only for one numerically insignificant entity, interstitial cystitis.

I am willing to make the statement to this Committee that there is no question concerning the effectiveness of DMSO. It is one of the few agents in which effectiveness can be demonstrated before the eyes of the observers. For instance, if we have patients appear before the Committee with edematous sprained ankles, the application of DMSO would be followed by objective diminution of swelling within an hour. No other therapeutic modality will do this.

If we have patients appear with acute bursitis unable to move a shoulder in any direction, the topical application of DMSO would be followed by a dramatic increase in the range of motion at the end of a half hour. If we have patients appear with chronic bursitis, the topical application of DMSO would be followed by a notable increase in the range of motion within a half hour.

If we have patients appear with fresh ecchymoses such as an early black eye, a topical application of DMSO would be followed by a reduction in this discoloration within one hour.

An NDA on DMSO for scleroderma was submitted almost three years ago. During this time we have revised the submission several times to meet decision delaying tactics. This NDA was turned down by the FDA. The FDA is currently considering whether to require additional months, or most probably years, before they approve this indication. These delays cause unnecessary suffering for thousands of Americans and possibly the loss by otherwise unnecessary amputation of fingers, toes, and limbs. This is an intolerable situation.

Dimethyl sulfoxide (DMSO) is a particularly promising treatment with injuries of the central nervous system (brain and spinal cord). Data from lower animals and man indicate that DMSO may be more important than any other pharmacologic agent in treating injuries to the brain and spinal cord.

With such a promising new medical application for DMSO, one might presume that we are satisfied and optimistic about the project's future. This is far from the truth. Results with CNS [central nervous system] accidents, to date, though dramatic and lifesaving, are not even fractionally different from multiple clinical findings with DMSO for other disorders.

Heretofore, every time we have concluded a clinical study demonstrating efficacy and safety with DMSO, we have been rewarded with a new, stabilized FDA position of confoundment. An obdurate barrier of bureaucrats housed in the offices of the FDA has shredded the data with their own unique methodology. In their house, supported by public funds, they play dangerous games—harmful games with truth, statistics, objectivity, ethics and the health and welfare of citizens of the U.S. If their policies with DMSO are an accurate barometer of their general procedures with food and drug policies, the Bureau itself may be a great hazard to the health of the people of this country.

Let me make a grim prediction concerning the fate of our CNS-DMSO projects. Unless responsibility for DMSO decisions is removed from the FDA or the FDA is subject to a radical change in management, despite the potential savings of tens of thousands of lives per year or prevention of permanent paralysis, post-CNS accident, FDA will continue to block public access to the drug for at least several years. Recall the so-called "historical" control to this matter—FDA has blocked other important medical usage of DMSO in man for more than 15 years.

The major question continues to be, has the public benefited, or has the public been harmed by the FDA blockade on approving DMSO. If DMSO had been truly a nostrum, or even worse, a drug associated with serious clinical toxicity, the public would have benefited by FDA actions. If, as overwhelming scientific evidence indicates, DMSO is a significant medical advance with minimal clinical toxicity, then the public has been and continues to be harmed by the FDA approach.

—Stanley W. Jacob, M.D.
Associate Professor
Department of Surgery
University of Oregon
Health Sciences Center

TESTIMONY OF ROBERT J. HERSCHLER
IN FAVOR OF HOUSE BILL NO. 88,
WASHINGTON STATE, FEBRUARY 17, 1981

This considered Bill states it to be an act related to health. The intent is to improve not only the health but the welfare of citizens of Washington State by legalizing prescriptive dimethyl sulfoxide (DMSO).

DMSO is a safe and effective drug that not only alleviates pain and suffering in man, but is the only known therapy for serious, debilitating diseases. DMSO is lifesaving where severe trauma is presented; oftentimes there is no adequate alternative therapy. In the next several years, Americans and all peoples of this world predictably will reflect on how and why the U.S. Food and Drug Administration was able to deny for so many years the safest and most broadly effective medicine yet provided by good science to this time in our hstory.

We are collecting the statements on DMSO, as in print, and provided by FDA since 1964. Our intent is to publish these with proper criticism. None are entirely truthful. One must learn that FDA is a political, not a science-oriented agency. FDA is an agency that needs dramatic change. Its Humpty-Dumpty policy makers sitting with ineptitude on their Rockville, Maryland, wall have made a shambles of drug research in the United States of America. I believe FDA has little or no intention of expediting further DMSO approval for human use. Their only defense to date has been that properly controlled studies have not been completed. False!

Furthermore, let us look at the result from perhaps overcontrolled studies this past decade. The drugs released as Ibuprofen, Sulindac, Fenoprofen Calcium, Oxyphenbutazone, Meclofenamate Sodium, Indomethacin, Tolmetin Sodium, Immunosuppressives, Gold Sodium Thiomalate, Aurothioglucose, etc., are symptomatic of a regulatory disease. Why must a drug be so toxic it can cause serious ocular toxicity in man, blood and lymph disorders, and the most serious side effect of all, death, at FDA-recommended dosages? Pity the patient that overdoses. DMSO causes none of these serious side effects.

At this time, FDA appears to believe that harsh tactics are called for to combat the opposition. They have recently tooled up their propaganda machinery to increase the output of misleading propaganda, and have initiated harassment tactics aganst scientists and support structures that provide new and factual evidence of DMSO's medical worth.

FDA, before any clinical data were forthcoming, determined that DMSO's drug use would be difficult for them to control and also feared that so many drug applications would be filed, it would overwork this lethargic bureaucracy. They sought any excuse to discredit DMSO and terminate clinical research. Eye changes in certain laboratory animals, at high dosage levels, over extended test periods caused changes in the index of refraction of the lens. Subsequent studies have shown these changes cannot be confirmed in man. Doses of up to 9 GM/KG × 18 months in the monkey, a truly massive challenge, elicited no exceptional toxicity findings, eye or otherwise.

In our boundary state, Oregon, new legislation is under consideration which will provide properly formulated DMSO to its citizens at approximately the following cost structure per 8-ounce bottle:

$1.00–$1.25 per unit fully packaged
$1.00–added state tax
 0.50–fund for research
 0.50–as profit and license fees to manufacturer, for a total of circa $3.00–$3.25 per unit wholesale.

It would be supplied to licensed pharmacies for prescriptive filling.

The reasons why FDA historically propagandized against and blocked DMSO studies in earlier years have now given way to a far more serious concern. FDA now knows that thousands of Americans die each year because they are denied DMSO therapy, tens of thousands are unnecessarily mutilated, and millions of our people suffer needless pain. FDA knows they are guilty of causing a disaster. The thalidomide tragedy resolved by a worldwide effort of science (*not FDA*) is but a molehill by comparison.

In my view, FDA should be subject to a thorough investigation of their mishandling of the entire DMSO question, and sanctions imposed where indicated.

The Government of Washington State must provide its people with access to properly formulated DMSO, by reason that the FDA has little or no intention of acting to this matter.

—ROBERT J. HERSCHLER

Index